3

2

Existential Neurosis

Existential Neurosis

E. K. Ledermann

M.D., M.R.C.Psych.
Physician, Royal London Homoeopathic Hospital;
Psychiatrist, Marlborough Day Hospital, London

LONDON
BUTTERWORTHS

ENGLAND: BUTTERWORTH & CO. (PUBLISHERS) LTD.
LONDON: 88 Kingsway, WC2B 6AB

AUSTRALIA: BUTTERWORTH & CO. (AUSTRALIA) LTD.
SYDNEY: 586 Pacific Highway, 2067
MELBOURNE: 343 Little Collins Street, 3000
BRISBANE: 240 Queen Street, 4000

CANADA BUTTERWORTH & CO. (CANADA) LTD.
TORONTO: 14 Curity Avenue, 374

NEW ZEALAND: BUTTERWORTH & CO. (NEW ZEALAND) LTD.
WELLINGTON: 26–28 Waring Taylor Street, 1

SOUTH AFRICA: BUTTERWORTH & CO. (SOUTH AFRICA) (PTY) LTD.
DURBAN: 152–154 Gale Street

Suggested UDC number: 616–891

ISBN: 0 407 17040 5

Printed in Great Britain by
Redwood Press Limited, Trowbridge, Wiltshire

Dedicated to my patients

Contents

Preface

The subject of this book is medical, but it is not only addressed to doctors, for its theme is of universal interest: the predicament of modern man who is liable to break down, unable to cope with life. Man is suffering from lack of faith, his symptoms take him to the doctor, but medical science cannot deal with his problem. My interpretation of the phenomenon of neurotic man is in terms of a personalistic existential ethic which is medically oriented.

I presented my ideas first in lectures and seminars as visiting professor to the Psychiatric Department at the University of Virginia in 1967 and I am now offering them to a wider public.

London

E. K. Ledermann

Symptoms

1

The Extent of Neurotic Suffering

Neurotic illness is causing severe suffering to contemporary man. The neurotic is unable to enjoy his life; he is anxious and tense, and this tension has adverse effects also on his physical health, affecting especially his blood pressure, his heart, his digestive organs, and his muscles. It interferes with his sleep and with his capacity to carry out physical and mental work. He gets tired and exhausted quickly, is depressed and irritable, feels insecure and unable to cope with life.

The prevalence of emotional disorder has been discovered by thorough questioning of a representative sample of the population. Such a survey was carried out by Anthony Ryle, a general practitioner in London, assisted by a psychiatric social worker and a consultant psychiatrist. Ryle has described his findings in a book entitled *Neurosis in the Ordinary Family.*[1]

Ryle found that 'some 30 per cent or so of the population . . . present with chronic or recurrent symptoms of emotional stress and tension. These are the more or less insecure, immature people with only partially-met dependent needs, whose adjustment to life is maintained only at the price of some restriction and of some symptoms.'[2]

Suffering is not confined to the neurotic, it also affects his surroundings, especially members of his family. A neurotic parent is inconsistent in the treatment of the children and also interferes with their development by trying to dominate them. Sons often react by an acting-out of their rebellion which is expressed in antisocial behaviour. Daughters are inhibited in their normal development.[3]

Ryle and his co-workers became convinced as the result of their study that a large proportion of these children were liable to be damaged or restricted in their further development. Assessing the chances of such a child attaining maturity and stability, the author concluded that '28 per cent of the children [in a disturbed family] . . . have a poor outlook'.[4]

With regard to emotional disturbances in children within the total population, Ryle quoted the following figures: a survey of 1,000 families in Newcastle showed that at least one in five of the child population was disturbed at the age of 11, and in a small Norwegian town, one quarter of the children aged 5–14 years gave evidence of a psychological disturbance. An American enquiry gave similar results: '20 per cent of the parents [of the families which were investigated] came from broken homes' and it was estimated that 'a similar proportion of the children [in this sample] will experience broken homes before they reach the age of 15'. Another author, Wardle, found that 31 per cent (perhaps more) of parents and 35 per cent of children had suffered that fate. The experience of a broken home in childhood is associated with neurosis in later life.[5]

In spite of marked improvement in the conditions under which people live and in spite of the intensive study of mental and emotional illness by a great many experts, neutotic illness is on the increase.

The rise of psychoneuroses affects all sections of the community. Surgeon Capt. Frank P. Ellis, Medical Officer in Charge, Royal Naval Medical School, told a meeting of the Chadwick Trust in London that remittent fevers and rheumatism, formerly common complaints in the navy, had disappeared, but that 'they had to deal with the appearance of psychoneuroses which were not shown in the health tables of a century ago'.[6]

Apart from the presence of emotional and psychosomatic symptoms, neurosis is evident from people's dependency on drugs which affect the nervous system. They cause serious suffering.

Alcohol is an example. 'It is estimated that there are about 100,000 acute alcoholics in England and Wales... Less acute alcoholics are probably three times as numerous... In Scotland alcoholism is the cause of admission to mental hospital of one patient in five.'[7] 'There are five million alcoholics in the USA and the disease is listed as the fourth worst for shortening life.'[8]

Dependency on smoking is another manifestation of neurosis. 'Half the population of England and Wales over the age of 16 are regular smokers and four fifths have had some experience of smoking, according to a survey of smoking habits and attitudes conducted for the Ministry of Health... The number of women who smoked was increasing and they were starting at an earlier age. Half the people who smoked either wanted to give it up or had tried to do so, but unsuccessfully... It was estimated that 22 per cent of former smokers (not severe addicts) had managed to give up the habit.'[9]

The harm to a person's physical health from smoking can be assessed from the findings of the Surgeon-General's Advisory Committee on

Smoking and Health: 'Cigarette-smoking, it [the Committee] has no doubt, is *causally* related to lung cancer in man and in importance outweighs all other factors. . .Cigarette-smoking is also judged to be a signficant factor in the causation of cancer in larynx in men, while a causal relationship also appears to be established between pipe-smoking and the development of cancer of the lip. . .Cigarette-smoking. . . is the most important of the causes of chronic bronchitis in the U.S.A., and for chronic broncho-pulmonary disease as a whole it is of much greater importance for the bulk of the population than atmospheric pollution or occupational exposure. . . In Great Britain much of this appears to be true also. . . In the U.S.A. deaths from coronary thrombosis and from arterioslerotic and degenerative heart disease rose from 273,000 in 1940 to 396,000 in 1950 and 578,000 in 1962. From the results of seven prospective studies the Committee shows the observed deaths of cigarette-smokers from coronary disease to be 70% in excess of those expected at the death-rate of non-smokers. . .While the Committee refrains from concluding that the association of cigarette-smoking with cardiovascular disease is one of cause and effect it does not hesitate to point out that it would be prudent to assume that, in fact, it is so.' The total increase of the death rate in the U.S.A. through smoking in men is estimated to be a 70 per cent increase, in women less.[10] Deaths caused by smoking in Britain have been estimated by Sir George Godber, Chief Medical Officer of Health, to amount to 100,000 a year. He called cigarette smoking the biggest avoidable menace to health.[11]

Alcohol and nicotine are the most important drugs which people who cannot cope with life prescribe for themselves. They are not called drugs, as they are not obtained from chemists. Doctors add enormously to the drugging of the neurotic population. According to W. Sargant 'most of the forty-three million NHS prescriptions for psychotropic drugs dispensed over a recent three-year period were to combat states of anxiety and tension. This total did not include the tranquillizers, sedatives and anti-depressants used in general and mental hospitals and also in the large additonal private practice of medicine and psychiatry.'[12] Sedative drugs carry the risk of addiction, whether they belong to the group of barbiturates or not.[13]

Addiction to opiates, amphetamines, marihauna, and hallucinogens has become news recently. The misery suffered by these addicts, most of them young people, is enormous, particularly if they cannot obtain heroin, if they have to rely on bigger and bigger doses of amphetamines to keep going, and if their LSD trip has gone wrong. Some suffer the agonies of psychotic breakdowns as the result of their drug experiences. In Great Britain and America the number of addicts is growing at a frightening rate, and so is their suffering. They use drugs to counteract their anxiety, depression, and apathy; Lady Frankau described addicts as follows: 'Addicted patients are asocial, inadequate, immature and unstable. They are selfish and self-centred without any interest in the welfare of others and are only concerned in their own problems. Their major problem is in the maintenance of the supply of drugs or the immediate gratification of their desire for drugs. They will resort to any means – however unreasonable or dangerous – to satisfy this insistent craving. They have failed to develop normal human relationships and are almost totally without concern for the distress they inflict on their relatives. They lack self-discipline, will-power or ambition, and avoid responsibility. They have a low threshold for pain or any form of discomfort and are unable to tolerate criticism or to bear frustration. Their personal relationships tend to become confined to other members of the drug addicts' world and thus they become social outcasts and very lonely people.'[14] Their loneliness is a measure of their suffering, and they become more lonely as they sink more and more deeply into their addiction. Their personalities crumble.

People who are emotionally disturbed are not only addicted to drugs, but also to food. Especially sugar and starch are eaten in large quantities to satisfy their craving for sympathy which is unfulfilled. They experience the agonies of finding their overweight bodies ugly and unacceptable. Their treatment is usually quite unsuccessful although, in contrast to the drug addicts, they make frequent attempts to be 'cured'. Such people do not only suffer psychological hardship, but also serious physical consequences. Diabetes, emphysema, atherosclerosis (causing coronary disease and peripheral arterial disease), gall-stones, and high blood pressure are conditions associated with obesity which is thus an important factor in shortening a person's life and which has become a nationwide problem in countries with a high standard of living.

Such is the extent of neurotic suffering.[15]

Diagnosis

2

Neurosis as a Scientific Phenomenon

UNCERTAINTY IN PSYCHIATRY

What sort of phenomenon is this wide spread condition called neurosis? By calling it a disease it becomes a disorder which medical science is expected to study and to treat. It is classed as an illness of the mind in correspondence to the illnesses of the body.

A. Ryle concluded his investigations of neurosis in the ordinary family by expressing his 'hope that an increasing proportion of the younger generation [of family doctors] may be able to accept psychiatry as a scientific and respectable branch of medicine'.[1]

There is no doubt that there is a very urgent need for family doctors to try to help the enormous number of neurotics who are under their care, but it does not follow that the phenomenon of neurotic illness is amenable to scientific treatment.

Accepting the scientific approach means that scientific knowledge must be available before success in treatment or in prevention can be expected. Many authorities admit that at present the medical profession fails to help the huge number of neurotic patients, and psychiatrists are themselves unsure in their approach.

A paper entitled 'Opinions on Psychotherapy: An Enquiry' revealed a state of great confusion in the minds of those who hold responsible positions as specialists in psychological medicine. The authors of the paper, R. M. Mowbray and G. C. Timbury, collected information from psychiatrists practising in Scotland and found that the responses to their questions 'showed wide variations of opinions and practice regarding the definition of the term [psychotherapy], the techniques used and the training thought to be desirable'.[2]

A variety of approaches may, of course, be beneficial for the patients and may be a sign of open-mindedness on the part of the doctors, but Mowbray and Timbury did not arrive at such favourable conclusion. To them, the current practice in psychotherapy suggested a state of 'arbitrariness'. They quoted another author, Colby, who had carried out a similar review in 1963 and had opened his report 'with the simple phrase "choas prevalis" '.[3]

The enquiry has revealed a most alarming position with regard to psychotherapy: 'Of the whole group, 60 [out of 100] stated that they had been formally trained in psychotherapy. . . Of the group of 60 respondents who had formal training only 30. . . said that their training was satisfactory. Of the 40 with no formal training only 6 expressed satisfaction.'[4] Thus out of one hundred psychiatrists only thirty-six considered their training as psychotherapists satisfactory. Such a situation would be unthinkable in physical medicine or surgery.

Satisfactory training in any form of medical treatment depends on a satisfactory theory from which the treatment follows. Psychiatry is without such firm foundation. According to Sir Aubrey Lewis, psychiatry is at present 'in much the same state as medicine was at the end of the eighteenth century', therefore it 'cannot be presented to the medical student as an adequate theoretical system or as a body of established and classified facts about causes, pathology, course and treatment of mental diseases'.[5] Thus we are waiting for knowledge, not just for the discovery of facts, but for the correct theoretical approach which would provide a framework for classification and for treatment. Comparing psychiatry with well-established sciences, Sir Aubrey Lewis wrote: 'We are not living through a period that marks a new epoch: there is no Galileo or Darwin, no Harvey or Newton, in psychiatry and psychology: nor – to put our aspirations on a more realistic plane – have there been discoveries during the last twenty years comparable to those that have signalled the growth of therapeutics and surgery in other medical fields.'[6]

Especially in a matter of such vital importance as the treatment of emotional disorders, a doctrinal standpoint is inexcusable, but Sir Aubrey Lewis finds that certain of his colleagues adopt such a standpoint with regard to such crucial factors as the mental constitution and the role played by the environment in these conditions. He himself sides with those to whom 'on sober review, such questions seem still largely unanswered', and he holds that 'the driving forces of human conduct, shaping our minds for good or ill, are recondite, and though everybody forms opinions and working hypotheses on these matters, many psychiatrists, on reflection, are ready to admit to much uncertainty and ignorance'.[7] My question is: is the scientific approach the correct approach, to gain knowledge of the 'driving forces of human conduct' on which mental health depends, and to treat the conditions which result from disturbances of such forces? Perhaps psychological medicine cannot hope to achieve the status which physical medicine occupies, and the waiting for a Galileo, Newton, or Darwin is in vain. We cannot take it for granted that these recondite forces can be known and that scientific hypotheses can be formulated and applied to the prevention and treatment of neurosis. While this specific illness is the subject of this book, it must be treated as an aspect of mental health in general and must be related to the fundamental problem of the knowability of the mind in health and in disease.

ENQUIRY INTO THE KNOWABILITY OF THE PSYCHE

Before we can decide whether knowledge of the healthy and of the sick mind can be obtained and can be incorporated in a scientific psychiatry, we have to define the criteria which are valid for scientific knowledge. Therefore we must start our enquiry by investigating the structure of science and must then apply the outcome of this investigation to psychiatry.

Tests for a science of the mind

In his essay entitled 'The Nature and Aim of Science', Ernest Nagel has given the following definition: 'science . . . is . . . directed to the attainment of systematic but reliable *knowledge*, so that its products are taken to be warranted *conclusions* about more or less extensive uniform conditions under which various kinds of events take place.'[8] The scientific enquiry rests on a presupposition: the scientific phenomena occur in an orderly fashion, they are *determined,* and the scientist's assumption of determinism is expressed in his aim 'to exhibit events and processes as instances of general laws and theories which formulate invariable patterns of relations between things'.[9]

The theories or hypotheses must be tested for their validity, and the testing involves the elimination of a counter-theory or counter-hypothesis which means that the scientist checks or controls his theoretical assumptions. 'The reliability of scientific conclusions is a function of the multiplicity and of the rigor of the controls to which such conclusions have been subjected.'[10] Individual phenomena are explained in the light of the particular theory, they are 'linked to each other in determinate ways by virtue of their place in some system of explanations'.[11]

The assumption of laws implies the assumption of causes which stand for the principle of necessity or determinism. We thus speak of causal laws.

Whereas the causal law asserts that one particular event is invariably associated with another event, the statistical law merely asserts that 'in a sufficiently long series of trials, the occurrence of one event is accompanied by the occurrence of a second event with an invariable relative frequency. Such laws... are not incompatible with a causal account of the facts they formulate'; they are used in 'areas of inquiry... in which the explanation of phenomena in terms of strictly universal causal laws is not likely to be feasible practically'. They are 'used as the proximate premises for the explanation and prediction of many phenomena'.[12]

The science of the body satisfies the conditions laid down by Nagel. The body is therefore an object of science and is knowable in terms of refutable theories. Laws are discoverable which enable doctors to treat the sick body and to prevent its illness. Although the physiology and the pathology of the body is not explained by a single theory – an infectious disorder is not known by means of the same concepts as a degenerative condition for instance – there is no contradiction in the different approaches to the body.

Contradictory views are held with regard to the functioning of the mind, and this division of psychiatrists initiated the enquiry into the knowability of the psyche. The object of the investigation is to test the tenets of each school for the validity of its theoretical structure and for its accountability of a patient's psyche. If the scrutiny should reveal that psychiatry cannot pass the test of a scientific discipline, it might disclose the reason for this failure and might point the way to a non-scientific interpretation of the mind.

We shall first examine the organic school of psychiatry. Its theoretical framework is derived from biological sciences, especially from neurophysiology and neuropharmacology.

Biological psychiatry

Neurophysiologists have established connections between the brain and the mind and have located certain parts of the brain which are associated with certain emotional conditions; for example, rage and fear can be produced in animals by stimulation of the amygdala, the hippocampal-cingulate system appears to be concerned with memory, and the hippocampus participates also in emotional responses. Neurologists have added to our knowledge of the significance of the brain for the mind: epileptic patients suffer from emotional disturbances and often from intellectual impairment, arteriosclerotic disease of the brain is manifest by deterioration of all the mental functions. Neuropharmacology can be applied in the treatment of emotional disturbances. Psychotropic drugs have proved most valuable in helping psychotics, and they also relieve neurotic suffering.

The theories of neurophysiology and neuropharmacology are scientifically sound, as they can be checked and refuted by counter-theories. Biological psychiatry is right in applying the knowledge which is gained from these theories, it treats the mind by treating the brain (with medicine, electric currents, or surgery).

The effects which different drugs have on the brain and the mind have been associated with different types of people. This research has led to the choice of the correct dosage. H. J. Eysenck found for instance that the brain cortex of extraverts is in a relatively inhibited state. These patients require therefore comparatively small amounts of a sedative such as sodium amytal, for quieting their minds, whereas introverts show the opposite condition of their brain and need therefore comparatively large doses of sodium amytal for calming. Eysenck postulated an 'extraversion-introversion continuum': psychopaths have the lowest threshold, then follow hysterics, 'mixed neurotics', anxiety states; obsessionals and reactive depressives showed high sedation thresholds. This theory has been confirmed by experiment.[13]

Although we know that certain parts of the brain are associated with certain mental functions, that certain diseases of the brain are accompanied by certain disturbances of the mind, and that certain types of people are characterized by certain responses of their brains to drugs, we are not entitled to conclude that a person's mind is knowable in terms of the science of the brain.

The splitting up of the personality into body and mind, as it was carried out by Descartes, is artificial, but the division has been useful in medicine where it has led to a distinction of physical and mental illnesses. Descartes' separation of two realms, of two entities, is misleading if it is supposed that they can both be equally known. Because doctors have gained knowledge of the brain and of associations of cerebral states with mental states, the assumption has been made that a bridge joining the two realms can be constructed. In fact, the mental realm is the sphere of subjective experience, of thought, will, and feeling. One objective manifestation of the mind is the personality which reveals itself to the mind of another person. This knowledge which people have of one another is, however, not scientific knowledge, as it is not conceptual-theoretical. Only man's physical realm is knowable, the cerebral part, for instance, in terms of neurophysiology and neuropharmacology.

The attempt to account for the mental realm in terms of the physical realm is a logical mistake, as each of these worlds are ultimate (although artificially created by the separation of the body-mind unity). As D. O. Hebb has said, 'explanation is a process of reducing one set of ideas to another... To explain how nervous impulses can be translated into mental experience is, in the words of the preacher, an attempt to unscrew the inscrutable'.[14]

We must conclude that the study of the brain does not provide us with the knowledge of the mind, that there is no theory of the mind which can be expressed in terms of cerebral (bodily) phenomena and which can be checked by a counter-theory. Although psychiatrists can make use of neurological knowledge in order to relieve the suffering of people's minds, they cannot know the mind by means of biological (organic) psychiatry.

Genetic psychiatry

Neurophysiology and neuropathology are sciences of the body and not of the mind, but there is a science which combines an account of bodily and mental events, the science of genetics, and we must enquire whether the mind is knowable in terms of this discipline.

Geneticists formulate laws which reveal the causal influence of heredity; they identify the genetic material in bodily constituents, in the chromosomes. Normal mental characteristics such as musical talent and abnormal mental conditions such as psychotic illnesses are thus accounted for. The role of heredity in neurosis has, however, been disputed.[15] Normal physical conditions, such as the shape of the nose, and abnormal physical states, such as certain types of anaemia, are also explained by this science.

Geneticists do not predict a particular person's mental (or physical) make up. Their laws do not apply to an individual human being, as they are statistical laws which determine the chances of an inherited trait occurring in subsequent generations.

Apart from the fact that the science of genetics is concerned only with the probability of inheritance, it makes no claim of providing knowledge of a mind as a whole, that is, of a human person; for it restricts itself to an investigation into such partial characteristics as mood vacillation, sexual tendencies, and intelligence. When studying psychiatric inherited conditions, geneticists take into account the possibility of biological determinants, for instance disturbances in brain functioning, even if their nature is only hypothetical. Examples are the two main mental illnesses, schizophrenia and manic-depressive psychosis. Genetic psychiatry thus incorporates the approach of biological psychiatry.[16]

The mind is not knowable as an addition of gene-specificities. They do not account for the part played by the environment and they fail to explain the fullness of psychic life, manifest in a healthy, creative personality or in an anxious, depressed or otherwise disturbed neurotic patient. We must now investigate the science of the psyche, psychology, which claims to provide such knowledge.

Psychological psychiatry

Psychology is not only concerned with the whole psyche, but also with single psychic phenomena, which are assessed for instance as patients' intelligence, their emotional status, and their response to treatment. Apart from these static estimations, there are dynamic theories. As biological medicine determines mechanisms of the body, so psychological medicine determines mechanisms of the mind, replacement of one feeling by another, projection, identification, introjection etc. Chains of association of ideas are also causal-deterministic conceptions which follow from the dynamic, scientific approach and which are of interest to the psychiatrist. None of these enquiries into particular phenomena are, however, relevant to our question of whether the mind as a whole can be known by means of a deterministic approach, whether a scientific theory is available to explain 'the driving forces of human conduct, shaping our minds for good or ill,' or whether all such theories are unscientific, irrefutable, and dogmatic.

There is dogmatism, if one human trait becomes the only trait which determines the psyche. Freudian psychology is such an example. Freudians claim that 'psychoanalysis alone is built upon scientific insight and that the therapy is also a research method affording further scientific insight that is not only useful in treating neuroses but that is also of more universal application'.[17] Freud's theory postulates that neurotic illness is a disturbance of a person's instinctual life, and the treatment of neurotic adults aims at the establishment of genital primacy through regulating their libidinal economics and thus enabling them to enjoy 'regular satisfaction'.[18] In this hypothesis all manifestations of the mind are interpreted in libidinal terms, and in this one-sidedness lies its metaphysical, dogmatic, irrefutable character.

Although the leaders of the different schools of psychological psychiatry have not provided us with scientific knowledge of the psyche, they have widened our conception of human nature. Freud has made us aware of the part played by unconscious sexual phantasies, motives, and feelings. (His followers differ from him and from each other in their interpretation of the unconscious.) Alfred Adler has opened our eyes to the implications of the striving for superiority and Jung has revealed to us the significance of the fundamental experiences which are shared by all men. All these contributions bear the stamp of absoluteness and their respective claims to truth cannot be settled scientifically.

The dilemma of psychological psychiatry was highlighted by Gordon W. Allport in the following sentences: 'Our assumptions regarding the nature of man range from the Adlerian to the Zilborgian, from the Lockian to the Leibnizian, from the Freudian to the Hullian, and from the cybernetic to the existentialist. Some of us model man after the pigeon, others view his potentialities as many splendored. And there is no agreement in sight.'[19] We are bound to add, nor can there ever be any agreement.

Patients suffer from the one-sidedness of particular psychological theories. In order to provide them with a full chance of being helped, two proposals have been made.

Eclecticism is the first suggestion; it consists in the selection of the theory which is correct for a particular patient. The choice could be made only by someone who owes no allegiance to a particular school, who is not convinced that his theory is the whole truth; for a Freudian will not select a non-Freudian approach, a Jungian a non-Jungian. Eclecticism sounds very broad minded, but it is difficult to see how it can be applied. Is the therapist to grant some of his patients the status of the pigeon and not others? Do any of the assumptions provide for the full potentialities of the person? If the therapist has not been analysed according to the rites of all the schools, he does not know the full measure of unconscious life.

The second proposal is the adoption of a comprehensive theory which combines all the features of human nature and which includes both scientific determinism and freedom. Allport's own system belongs to this class. It comprises exchange of matter and energy, safeguarding of biological and psychological equilibrium, consideration of libidinal pleasure, striving for power and leadership, readiness to perform one's duty, recognition of the need for meaning in life, and consideration of the significance of cultural, social, and family influences on the individual.[20]

H. Cantril has offered a 'human design' which claims to account for the following human needs: survival, security, order and certainty, enlargement and enrichment of satisfactions, hope, striving, choices, exercise of will to act, experience of identity, integrity, worthwhileness and values.[21] Such a comprehensive view does not provide scientific knowledge of the psyche because it includes both deterministic and libertarian elements.

The fault of Allport's open system consists in its failure to subordinate the deterministic biological, psychological, and sociological factors to man's capacity for facing their significance for the meaning of his life. Cantril's design is supposed to be 'genetically built-in' and lists 'the appetitive systems' (which man shares with the higher animals), propelling him and them 'to seek satisfying and pleasurable experiences' together with those systems which constitute a protection from threatening and unpleasant experiences.[22] In addition, the design includes man's ethical endowments which demand of him the confrontation of needs and experiences, the striving for a personal design of his life, and a refusal to be propelled by genes or appetites. The moral implication which is inherent in Allport's and Cantril's approaches demonstrates the fallacy of scientific psychological psychiatry. By their acknowledgement of human freedom, they have pointed to a non-deterministic interpretation of the mind.

Behaviouristic psychiatry

Certain psychiatrists have claimed that they can provide a deterministic explanation of the psyche solely by reference to the behaviour of the body. They are the behaviouristic psychiatrists. The underlying theory assumes that 'the occurrence of a psychic state in a body is always accompanied by certain overt and publicly observable behaviors. . .of that body; that such overt behaviors (including verbal responses) constitute a sufficient basis for grounding conclusions about the entire range of human experience; and that observation of such overt behavior is not only the sole source of information anyone has concerning other men's experiences and actions, but also provides generally more reliable data for conclusions even about an individual's own character and capacities than is supplied by introspective analyses of psychic states.'[23]

Behavioural psychiatry can be refuted by the argument which Charles Taylor set out in his book *The Explanation of Behaviour*. As he has pointed out, observation cannot yield knowledge of behaviour, for one can observe only movements of the body, but what counts are actions, and these are unobservable; for their explanation one requires a teleological explanation, which presupposes the anti-behaviouristic assumption of a purposeful mind. Two of Taylor's examples illustrate this vital point: one cannot understand a dog who wants food from the movements of its body, only from the action of snapping at the meat, nor can one understand people when they shake hands in terms of the movements of their arms, but only in terms of a meaningful action of their whole personalities.[24]

The need for the teleological explanation of behaviour is also evident in the case of learning and unlearning which play the fundamental part in behaviouristic psychiatry; neurotic behaviour is interpreted as being due to reception of the wrong stimuli and the treatment consists in the application of the 'appropriate' stimuli.

As Taylor has shown, the analytical stimulus-response molar theory is unable to account for learning, because learning involves discrimination, a mental act of cognition, a teleological process.[25] Animals and men explore their environment and learn to orientate themselves, to cope with whole situations.[26]

Ignoring the methodology which excludes the psyche, behavioural psychiatrists use psychic stimuli in order to extinguish neurotic responses. For instance, patients who are terrified of cats are told to imaging seeing a cat in the distance which is gradually lessened until they are 'desensitized' and can bear the actual sight of a cat. Whatever the practical results of such treatment may be, they cannot be explained by the behaviouristic theory, as the feared object means something to the patient and does not constitute an isolated psychic stimulus.

The psyche is not knowable in terms of behaviouristic determinism, the behaviour of men and of animals is in fact not behaviouristic, but is purposive and expresses itself in the freedom of actions. Men also possess moral freedom which is tested by the situations in which they find themselves, for instance by a neurotic illness (the phobic patient is expected to show his courage by facing the frightening experience).

Nosological psychiatry

Even if a patient's mind is not knowable in terms of the responses to isolated mental or physical stimuli, or of a thoery of human nature, is it knowable as the bearer of a disease? Nosological psychiatry implies the acceptance of such a view, and we must investigate its claim.

The nosological approach takes the scientific status for granted, it thus begs our question. The uncertainty amongst psychiatrists which gave rise to our enquiry cannot be settled by accepting the scientific naming of diseases of the mind as evidence for the scientific status of psychiatry.

J. G. Scadding has clarified the implications of nosology. As he has said, by naming diseases, 'we are referring to the whole complex of abnormal phenomena observed in a group of individuals selected because they present some stated common abnormality'.[27] Ryle informed us of the common abnormality of the neurotic patients: they 'present with chronic or recurrent symptoms of emotional stress and tension [and] are the more or less insecure, immature people with only partially-met dependent needs, whose adjustment to life is maintained only at the price of some restriction and of some symptoms'.[28]

By following the nosological approach, the psychiatrist registers the features which make up the illness, but he does not thereby understand the disease as his method is only descriptive and not dynamic, and therefore is not explanatory. The name neurosis, with its sub-divisions such as hysteria, obsessional-compulsive illness, anxiety states, and so on, does not refer to a testable scientific theory as for instance the name tuberculosis points to a complex of abnormal phenomena which are interpreted in terms of the testable aetiological, bacteriological hypothesis.

The designation of a condition such as neurosis as distinct from a psychosis (such as schizophrenia) is important, as the two names indicate distinct forms of suffering. The dis-ease of the mind is fundamentally different from the dis-ease of the body, as the mind stands for a whole personality suffering from a mental or physical dis-ease.

The nosological, the behaviouristic, the psychological, the genetic, and the biological psychiatric schools all fail to give a scientific account of a patient's total psyche. We must now examine the approach which takes as its starting point society and must enquire whether the psyche can be known in terms of its social surroundings.

Social psychiatry

The investigation into behaviouristic psychiatry revealed that the mind expresses itself by purposeful activity, by the striving for goals. The neurotic person, we found, suffers from a disability to cope with life, that is, from a weakness in striving which affects society, apart from himself.

The capacity to strive is a moral quality, as it involves the recognition of a duty; the neurotic fails to perform his duty towards himself and towards the group in which he lives. Although we cannot derive a patient's neurosis from a set of social events, we can define under what social circumstances his neurotic inability is likely to get worse and when it is liable to improve. On this knowledge depends his social treatment.

Social psychologists have studied the group dynamics which are relevant to our problem. Dorwin Cartwright for instance has given a summary of this subject in a paper, entitled 'Achieving Change in People: Some Application of Group Dynamics Theory'. His conclusions are that changes in individuals (whether of behaviour, of attitude, beliefs or values), depend on the group to which he belongs, as his aspirations, his loves and hates, his self-confidence or self-respect are 'highly determined' by his social milieu.[29]

In Cartwright's paper three ways of effecting a change are mentioned. Firstly, the group must be used 'as a medium of change', secondly the group itself must become 'the target of change', which means that its standards, atmosphere, hierarchical composition have to be considered.

Thirdly, special agents have to be employed to bring about the desired result, a committee or some form of new leadership are the vital factors.[30]

The non-deterministic, that is, non-scientific, nature of the three conditions becomes evident from their elaboration: the effective use of the group depends upon the closeness of the relationship between the people, the therapeutic atmosphere of the group requires the contribution of all the members (who have to be in sympathy with each other), and the prestige of a leader involves strength of character and reliability. Cartwright emphasizes the need for sharing of responsibility and for communication.

These basic principles have been put into operation in hospitals which are run as therapeutic communities. They rely on the moral qualities of their members, of staff and patients alike.

There is a sharing of responsibility for behaviour on a ward by all the patients and there is a renunciation of the authoritarian structure of the hospital, of the traditional hierarchical placing of doctors, nurses and patients. The staff and the patients acquire new self-images. Emotional difficulties of the staff are frankly faced and their role-relationships and involvements are clarified. Unconscious factors, fears, guilt, and remorse are recognized. Maxwell Jones, a pioneer in community psychiatry, has described the effects of this social treatment on patients as follows: 'In a ward where patients have had experience of responsible roles and are strongly identified with treatment aims, they will come to the aid of the night nurse in the event of disturbed behaviour, instead of leaving it entirely to her to deal with. In this context also, one finds patients are more able to bear with highly disturbed behaviour among their peers because the community meetings have helped them to understand the meaning of such behaviour and have given them a better idea of how to relate in a helpful way to a disturbed member. The daily examination of social interaction and difficulties on the unit means that the patients become aware of many of the factors which lie behind behaviour and learn a great deal about each other's problems.'[31]

In accordance with the professional tradition, Maxwell Jones finds a scientific, that is, deterministic basis for his practice of social psychiatry. He agrees with Jurgen Ruesch who 'describes social psychiatry as the product of a union between psychiatry and the social disciplines' and who stresses the contribution of 'the disciplines of sociology and anthropology, of epidemiology and ecology, and of preventive and therapeutic medicine'.[32]

Maxwell Jones is, however, careful not to commit himself; in order to give social psychiatry the widest definition, he prefers to keep this discipline elastic and to 'include [in it] all social, biological, educational, and philosophical considerations'[33] in order to give social psychiatry a full chance to develop. Such caution is in line with the empirical British tradition, but it does not promote progress. The basis of this approach is clear. Social psychiatry is founded on ethics and is, therefore, not a deterministic scientific discipline, although the knowledge of social, biological, and other sciences is relevant to the appreciation of the factors which have to be faced by the members of the therapeutic community.

The word morale occurs in Maxwell Jones' publications, but the term moral is avoided. This shyness was foreign to the psychiatrists of the Victorian era who unashamedly provided 'moral treatment' for their patients. The difference between their ethical conception and the moral philosophy which emerges from our enquiry lies in the roles assigned to the therapist and the patient. The Victorian psychiatrist regarded the mental patients 'as normal people who had lost their reason as a result of having been exposed to severe psychological and social stresses. These stresses were called the moral causes of insanity, and moral treatment aimed at relieving the patient by friendly association, internal discussion of his difficulties and the daily pursuit of purposeful activity.'[34] The underlying assumption is that the patient is a recipient of the treatment which must be provided for him, as he has been deprived of the moral qualities that enable normal people to cope with life. Our view is that the patient and those 'normal' people who look after him have the moral task of understanding each other and of facing the conflicts which are responsible for mental breakdowns. Therefore patients and staff are both active participants in the treatment. The very considerable success of the 'moral treatment' which psychiatrists carried out more than one hundred years ago, without the use of drugs and of other scientific aids, is a considerable credit to them and to their own moral stamina. It can be an inspiration to the present generation of doctors and should encourage them to consider the ethical implications of their practice, especially when dealing with the widespread sufferings of neurotic people.

Functional determinism in psychiatry

The moral basis of the therapeutic community is denied by those who subscribe to functional determinism. This application of the functional theory postulates that social systems tend to maintain themselves and that the stability of a social group is the result of an innate reciprocity of its members. Functional determinists assume that there is an automatic dynamism of interaction which makes each person honour his obligations to the other, all being moved by the feeling of mutual indebtedness. According to functionalism, people do not feel obliged to take responsibility for their action because their conscience demands such a conduct, nor are they free to decide what action to take, but 'the norm of reciprocity' is the determining factor governing human activity. E. Nagel has examined this theory of functionalism critically. He has pointed out that the theory rests on certain prerequisites which it fails to justify. Quoting Talcott Parsons' view that a social system has 'a persistent order' or undergoes 'an orderly process of developmental change',[35] Nagel points out that functionalists treat the social system as a unit, like a biological organism. This organismic assumption is, however, not justified. In biological structures we require the deterministic teleological conception in order to account for the survival of the organism; this elementary notion of survival does not, however, apply to social organisms, as they do not literally die.[36]

In the case of the hospital community, it is obvious that no natural basic stability causes all members to act in the functional-reciprocal manner. In fact, it requires extraordinary efforts by all concerned to achieve a measure of stability which, if it comes about, is greatly to the credit of the members of this community. Only by taking the moral motivations of the people in a community for granted, can we conclude that the system possesses a natural inherent tendency to maintain itself.

Apart from its teleological use, functionalism stands for formal interdependency. This is the meaning of function in a physical system where the term signifies 'relations of dependence or interdependence between two or more factors (or "variables")'.[37]

R. W. Angel applied the concept of function as employed in physical sciences to the psyche and asserted that 'psychic determinism may be defined without reference to causality by using the mathematical concept of function'.[38]

Angel's argument is fallacious. There is no doubt that one person is dependent on another, and that one's mental processes are dependent on one's bodily (especially cerebral) processes; such functional analysis does not, however, prove that the psyche as a whole is a system like a physical system which can be accounted for by the interaction of its variables.

Phenomenological psychiatry

Because of its ethical dimension, the psyche cannot be explained in terms of any scientific theory. Apart from conceptual knowledge, there is yet another form of understanding which is based on intuition or empathy. We must now examine its application to psychiatry which is called phenomenological psychiatry. Wilhelm Dilthey has characterized this approach as follows: 'On the basis of projection, this transposition, arises the highest form in which the totality of mental life can operate in the understanding – that of reproducing or reliving. . . Reliving means creating along the lines of events. . . Every vivid imaginative presentment of a milieu and an outward situation stimulates a reliving process in us. And fancy can strengthen or weaken the emphasis upon the attitudes, forces, feelings, strivings, lines of thought which are contained in our lives, and in this way can reproduce any other person's mental life.'[39]

Karl Jaspers, who studied under Dilthey, applied the intuitive approach to the subjective experiences of patients and called it 'understanding psychology' which he described in these words: 'Psychic events "emerge" out of each other in a way we understand. Attacked people become angry and spring to the defence, cheated people grow suspicious. The way in which such emergence takes place is understood by us, *our understanding is genetic.* Thus we understand psychic reactions to experience, we understand the development of passion, the growth of an error, the content of a delusion and dream; we understand the effects of suggestion, an abnormal personality in its context or the inner necessities of someone's life. Finally we understand the patient, how the patient sees himself and how this mode of self-understanding becomes a factor in his psychic development.'[40]

The intuitive grasp of genetic understanding does not lend itself to generalizations, to the formulation of objective laws which are the hallmark of conceptual-theoretical science. Jaspers' phenomenological approach in its original form applies only to an individual person, to the 'inner necessities' of a particular subjective world which it characterizes without interfering with the freedom of its spontaneity.

Other psychiatrists introduced into the subjective, phenomenological framework the objective classification of psychiatry. They have analysed and structured the worlds of schizophrenics, manic-depressives, hysterics, compulsive-obsessionals, and others. Minkowski for instance developed 'structural analysis' which was 'to define the basic disturbance (trouble générateur), from which one could deduce the whole content of consciousness and the symptoms of the patients'.[41]

The structural investigation of inner realms has revealed for instance that melancholic patients do not experience the stream of time as a drive forward, but as stagnation. The basic pathology in the schizophrenic world was found to consist in the 'loss of vital contact with reality'.[42]

The worlds of mental patients have been reconstructed from their basic constituents. The experience of time as lived time (in contrast to astronomical and biological time), the experience of space as oriented space and attuned space (in contrast to geometrical space), the experience of substance or matter (in contrast to chemical matter) and of causality as fate (in contrast to scientific determinism) form the main categories. They are all relevant for the way in which a person orientates himself in his world. Distortions in these fundamental experiences constitute deviations from the normal pattern of perception. The therapist must ascertain such data, as they are essential for the understanding of his patient.

Ellenberger singled out the experience of time as the factor which makes life either meaningful or empty. 'What we call the feeling of "the meaning of life" ', he said, 'cannot be understood independently of the subjective feeling of experienced time. Distortions of the feeling of time necessarily result in distortions of the meaning of life. Normally, we look upon the future not only for itself but also for compensating and correcting the past and the present. We reckon on the future for paying our debts, achieving success, enjoying life, becoming good Christians. Wherever the future becomes empty, as with manics and certain psychopaths, life is a perpetual gamble and the advantage of the present minute is taken into consideration; wherever the future is inaccessible or blocked, as with the depressed, hope necessarily disappears and life loses all meaning.'[43]

The above quotation reveals the deterministic outlook. The science of phenomenology which investigates patterns of subjective experience, is linked to the science of biology which investigates patterns of objective bodily phenomena. For instance, the appreciation of time has been found to depend on cellular metabolism and can be altered by drugs which affect the metabolism.[44] Tactile experiences depend on the state of the nerves which conduct stimuli to the brain. Tactile, visual, and auditory data form the important elements of a person's inner world and are related to cerebral structures and functions. Therefore a neurological examination of a patient is relevant for the appreciation of his experiential world.

Once the premise of phenomenological determinism has been accepted, patients are understood as living the lives of melancholics, hysterics, schizophrenics, and of other mental disorders. The distortions in their experience of time, space, causality, and matter are discovered as typical for the type of world to which they belong. The deterministic framework of the approach denies the individual his or her own world and existence. Like the other systems of psychiatry, phenomenological deterministic psychiatry cannot grasp the mind of a person.

Outcome of the enquiry into the knowability of the psyche

By classifying patients' worlds in nosological terms, phenomenological psychiatry accepts the deterministic framework of nosological psychiatry. By linking experience with cerebral events, the phenomenologist objectifies subjective experience in objective, biological terms. Although it was admitted that the mind depends on the brain for its functioning, knowledge of the brain was not accepted as knowledge of the mind. The freedom of individual mental life, apart from the genetic, neurological, and nosological frameworks, was postulated. This freedom is the freedom of a person in his own right who is not just the bearer of a disease, of a nervous system, and a set of genes.

The investigation into behavioural psychiatry revealed the fallacy of the underlying stimulus-response theory. Empirical observation of behaviour disclosed the fact that higher animals and human beings do not behave in a 'molar' fashion, but act according to a purpose which is conceived by their minds. The critique of the behaviouristic theory thus pointed to the freedom of action, of consciousness of a whole psyche. While the animal and man explore their environment and pursue their goals in an individual manner which cannot be accounted for by any natural law, man must be credited with a freedom which is not shared by the animal, with the freedom of accepting responsibility for his action, that is, with moral freedom.

The significance of responsibility became more evident when social psychiatry was examined, as responsibility plays in the vital role in society and is of crucial importance for the practice of community psychiatry, which, however, acknowledges also the deterministic aspects of social life.

To sum up: the psyche is not knowable in terms of a psychiatry which is based on scientific determinism. The neurotic person, like the 'normal' man, must face the responsibilities of his life to the best of his ability and must not leave his treatment to the scientific experts. His freedom is limited by all the factors which are studied scientifically, by the bodily and psychic mechanisms, the genetic endowment, the social circumstances, and the type of his illness. All these elements do not, however, negate his freedom, but represent a challenge to his freedom. Neurosis is not a scientific, but a moral phenomenon.[45]

3

Neurosis as a Moral Phenomenon

NEUROSIS AS A MANIFESTATION OF MAN'S MORAL CRISIS

Psychiatrists and the general population have to face the fact which has emerged from the foregoing enquiry. They have to interpret the symptoms and signs of neurosis in liberterian and not in deterministic terms. In order to clear the way for this orientation, we have to appreciate the power which the deterministic approach has on human minds; it stands for necessity and, in medicine, for the scientific laws which govern health and which explain illness. We have to realize that determinism has no claim to universal validity and to absolute truth. It is itself a necessary presupposition for the building up of scientific knowledge.

//Neurosis must be understood as a manifestation of man's moral crisis. This exposition has been accepted by a number of psychiatrists. Jung, for instance, made the following observation: 'About a third of my cases are suffering from no clinically definable neurosis, but from the senselessness and emptiness of their lives.' He recognized the significance of this statement when he wrote: 'It seems to me that this [suffering] can well be described as the general neurosis of our time.'[1]

Viktor E. Frankl has confirmed Jung's views. To Frankl, 'this striving to find a meaning in one's life is. . . regarded as the primary motivational force in man'.[2] He has pointed out that the frustration of the will to meaning leads to noogenic neuroses which he found to exist in 55 per cent of patients attending the neurological and psychotherapeutic clinics and of the medical and nursing staff.[3]

D. R. G. McInnes reported similar findings at the Annual Meeting of the British Medical Association in 1963. His patients were Oxford undergraduates whose 'breakdowns had become a matter not only of medical but of public interest'. He remarked that 'there were a considerable number of student patients whose trouble was not capable of formal diagnosis and who presented mainly with work and social difficulties, or with psycho-sexual problems. A characteristic feature of the group was the presence of a persistent feeling of pointlessness and futility. These students were unable to organize their lives or to establish goals towards which they might move. Their affective state had been likened to that of early schizophrenia but they were certainly not schizophrenic and did not become so.' McInnes discovered that these young people demanded a 'credo' from him and concluded 'this therapeutic situation epitomized the challenge of our time'.[4] How has this situation arisen?

In his book *Diagnosis of Our Time* the sociologist Karl Mannheim threw light on modern man's situation and explained why so many people feel life to be pointless and futile and why they suffer from nervous breakdowns.[5]

In the first chapter of his book, Mannheim stressed the influence of new social factors. Modern man's life is *planned*. 'The main changes we are witnessing to-day can ultimately be traced to the fact that we are living in a Mass Society.' This new form of social life manifests itself in certain forms of government policies: 'Government of the masses,' Mannheim pointed out, 'cannot be carried on without a series of inventions and improvements in the field of economic, political and social techniques' and he defined social techniques as 'the sum of those methods which aim at influencing human behaviour and which, when in the hands of the Government, act as an especially powerful means of social control'.[6]

It is obvious that the conditions of life have changed rapidly and are still changing in the direction characterized by Mannheim. The question is: why do people break down?

R. Dubos' answer is: because many cannot adapt themselves to the new situation. His view is that 'the marginal man' can tolerate a certain amount of disturbance, but 'is likely to break down when the extent and rate of change exceed his adaptive potentialities' and the author expects that 'for this reason mental diseases are likely to become more apparent in areas undergoing rapid cultural transitions, and this means a large part of the world'.[7]

Dubos described some of the features which give rise to mental breakdowns. 'The efficiency of industrial production is creating a pathology of boredom', the technological advance has deprived the individual of 'intimate participation in the creative activities of his group, [which] constitutes a much-needed sense of fulfilment... modern man has acquired the economic power to own things, but these are anonymously produced'.[8]

Doctors must recognize anonymity and lack of opportunities for creative activities as intolerable for man's self-respect and dignity, hence the breakdowns, caused by the lack of the much-needed sense of fulfilment, are a moral phenomenon, a protest against such conditions.

But is modern man, especially the youth, not encouraged to express his individuality? Efficiency of working conditions provides people with much leisure. Industrial societies 'enjoy material wealth and have the most effective social legislation', as Dubos remarked in his *Mirage of Health.* Why then do we find 'the highest rates of drug addiction, suicide, and death from violence' in the United States, Switzerland, Denmark, and Australia?[9]

Karl Mannheim provided the answer to this question: people are not only suffering from a lack of opportunities for expressing themselves, but much more from an uncertainty of values which can guide them in their expressions. Human society is disintegrating through a lack of values. As Karl Mannheim said: 'In a society where disintegration has proceeded too far, the paradoxical situation arises that education, social work and propaganda, notwithstanding highly improved techniques, become less and less efficient because all values that could guide them tend to evaporate.'[10]

Mannheim drew a very pertinent conclusion from his observation: 'What is the use,' he asked, 'of developing exceedingly skilful methods of propaganda and suggestion, new techniques of learning and habit-making, of conditioning, de-conditioning and re-conditioning, if we do not know what they are for? What is the good of developing child guidance, psychiatric social work and psychotherapy if the one who is to guide is left without standards? Sooner or later everyone becomes neurotic, as it gradually becomes impossible to make a reasonable choice in the chaos of competing and unreconciled valuations.'[11]

These sentences were written in 1942. During the intervening years, many psychiatric papers have been published and many clinics for psychiatric patients have been opened. The techniques of learning and conditioning to which Mannheim referred in 1942 have become some of the latest advances in psychotherapy. The implications of this form of treatment will be discussed in a later part of this book; at this point of the enquiry, it is important to realize that the essential trouble with the neurotic patient is a moral crisis and not a lack of opportunities in his surroundings or a lack of adaptability. By misinterpreting his situation, the therapist makes a wrong diagnosis, and it is a well-recognized principle in medicine that for the prescription of correct treatment the correct diagnosis is essential.

To the sociologist Mannheim, man's crisis had social causes. To him the variety of social values brought about conflicts which became unbearable: Christianity versus Marxian Materialism, craftsmanship versus mass production, obedience as a principle in education versus freedom of expression, authority in government control versus a policy of laisses-faire – these are some of the major antagonisms which he identified as the causes of the disturbances in the process of valuation.

A change in social norms and in ideologies can be unsettling to people. Children feel insecure if their parents and teachers have no definite principles. The loss of religious faith is the most profound cause for unsettlement, as it amounts to a loss of faith in a transcendental power. The individual person loses faith in himself under such conditions, and this loss brings about a nervous breakdown in those who are not strong enough to stand alone.

The ultimate test for preserving one's wholeness is, however, not whether one can endure a change in one's social pattern or even a lack of faith in God. The ultimate test is whether man can discover his moral strength to deal with his challenge. We shall now enquire into his potential to obtain help from systems expounded by traditional moral philosophers.

TRADITIONAL MORAL PHILOSOPHIES

Moral philosophers formulate theories in which they define value. They base their formulations on human experience on which they reflect and they arrive at definitions of such moral concepts as good, right, ought, duty and their opposites.

Bertrand Russell has pointed out that 'ethics is necessary because men's desires conflict'.[12] According to him, the conflict may be between egoistic and altruistic desires or between opposing ideologies.

There are sceptics who deny the theoretical validity of any moral standards; to them, moral judgements have no significance. Others base their systems on the concept of moral emotions and stress that the expressions of approval and disapproval voiced by society are the decisive element in the adoption of ethical standards. A further group deduces ethics from the evolution of the human race. Some writers make the experience of pleasure the criterion for right and wrong, but add the proviso that the happiness of the individual must not be attained at the cost of the unhappiness of others. Happiness is a feeling, an affect. To certain philosophers, this concept is too subjective, they base their judgement on objective standards: although pleasure may be desired by men, it is not necessarily desirable. Man's moral interest lies in defining what is right and what his duty is.

Goodness appears to some authors a metaphysical absolute which for the religious person is represented by God. The metaphysical theorists believe in a moral order of a spiritual kind and in man's obligation to realize his spiritual self. Value theories become idealistic theories, and the individual is expected to respond to the spiritual order. How is man to recognize the intrinsic good? The answer is: through intuition which is inherent in conscience; thus the right is apprehended as self-evident, and man's duty is clear: to strive for those aims which conscience recognizes as good.[13]

These different philosophies cannot be integrated within one system. Each theory reflects a certain attitude which its holder can defend against an opponent on purely theoretical grounds. The writers are not concerned with the consequences which arise from their moral theories. The traditional moral philosopher is not interested in the solution of the moral crisis and does not accept any responsibility towards his fellow men who suffer from the noogenic neurosis. We have to seek help from those thinkers who set out to provide an answer to man's predicament, to his lack of faith.

HUMANISTIC ETHICS

Some of those who have lost their faith in religion have postulated a faith in man, called humanism. The secular humanists are rationalists, full of trust in the ratio which has brought about the development of science.

Certain practical implications of the humanist philosophy were discussed by M. T. Hindson. He said: 'We believe, for example, that humanism should make us more unselfish and socially-minded, but there is a gap between the doctrine and the life which has not been systematically bridged.' He then described the material from which this bridge is to be constructed and the areas which it is supposed to join: 'From the mass of psychological and religious data which exists, it should be possible to construct a bridge, to build up a logic of feeling which would fulfil itself in unselfish behaviour.'[14] According to this author, the project has not been carried out because of 'the immensity of the universe and our own limitations of knowledge'.[15]

Hindson is mistaken: limitations of knowledge have nothing to do with the religious data which belong to a spiritual-moral order, a logic of feeling is self-contradictory, as feelings do not follow a logical course. Psychological data would form part of a deterministic science of the mind, which by its nature cannot be joined to religion.

Lance L. Whyte outlines another humanistic approach which also bears the marks of scientific rationalism. According to him, we require a broadened science for 'a real understanding of life, and therefore also of man. In other words, a humane science would show man the right way to think in order to understand nature and life, including himself'.[16]

A 'unified science' is utopian, for a science is limited to a field for which a certain set of concepts apply. In many endeavours, for instance in warfare, physical, biological, and sociological sciences are combined, although not unified in a single science. Such a combination provides no real understanding of life and does not make man truly human. It is naive of the rationalistic humanists to think that a humane science can be constructed and that man can learn wisdom by acquiring scientific knowledge. Wisdom is a quality of the human character which entails soundness of judgement in an intelligent and moral sense. Scientific knowledge must be subordinated to ethics if humaneness is to be achieved. An ethic can therefore not be based on scientific rationalism.

Some rationalistic humanists do not rely on science, but are led by the rational principle to a philosophy in which planning of happiness for all and efficiency play dominant parts. Erich Fromm belongs to this group. His humanistic ethics is of particular interest to us, as it claims to be applicable to our subject, to the problem of neurosis.

Fromm defines humanistic conscience and its aims as follows: 'humanistic conscience is knowledge within oneself, knowledge of our respective success and failure in the art of living' and 'the goal of humanistic conscience is productiveness and, therefore, happiness, since happiness is the necessary concomitant of productive living'.[17] Happiness is to be achieved therefore through 'the full development of productiveness'.[18]

Fromm's humanistic ethics is thus hedonistic. It associates with happiness all the things that people so much desire: 'increase in vitality, intensity of feeling and thinking' as well as productiveness.[19] There are the pleasures which are derived from the fulfilment of physiological needs which bring about 'the happiness of satisfaction', and there is the 'irrational pleasure' which is derived from the fulfilment of 'irrational desires', the neurotic desires which are concerned with the removal of painful tension. Fromm holds, however, that the happiness which is to be expected from liberation of tension is only temporary, the need is only mitigated and it points to 'pathological functioning' and to 'fundamental unhappiness'. The trouble, we are told, is that irrational strivings are all 'based on scarcity, on the lack of productiveness and inner security'. In contrast to this unproductive state, he affirms, the 'productive love', 'a phenomenon of abundance', the test for human maturity which brings joy and happiness.[20]

Fromm disagrees with those hedonists who take the achievement of pleasure to be an easy thing; to him, the development of full productiveness is man's most difficult task, hence his humanistic ethics, postulating happiness and joy 'as its chief virtues', makes great demands on man. The normal person 'possesses in himself the tendency to develop, to grow, and to be productive', but in the neurotic, we are told, there is 'a conflict between the inherent productive powers and those forces which block their development'. The failure to achieve the maturity of a developed and integrated personality represents 'a moral problem', present in every neurosis.[21]

Fromm illustrates his ethical-therapeutic approach by giving the example of a man who suffered from giddiness, from a neurotic symptom, interpreted as the protest of his better self against the betrayal of his views in his professional life as a teacher. We are asked to believe that the successful treatment brought about a victory of the 'basically moral personality', and this resulted in a growth of 'productivity' and in 'happiness'.[22]

But supposing the man, following his conscience, resigned from his position; supposing he held views which were unacceptable to the authorities, could not have remained a teacher, and that these views had landed him in prison, would he still have been happy and would he have achieved a growth of 'productivity' of his personality? He would hardly have experienced 'increase of vitality', he might have had intense feelings and thoughts but these are likely to have been intensely bitter, and he would have missed the joy of 'abundance'.

The linking of ethics with happiness is a fallacy. A moral action produces the satisfaction of a good conscience, but man cannot achieve good conscience if he aims at the feeling of satisfaction through his actions. The neurotic whose life feels empty may try desperately to fill it with pleasure and happiness, but his efforts will be in vain.

Although Fromm is correct when he states that 'every neurosis represents a moral problem', the problem is not solved by the humanist conscience which tells the neurotic to be more productive, nor is his wretched state due to his submission to others, as Fromm holds.[23] It is true that all men want happiness, which means not a temporary, partial state of some pleasure or enjoyment, but, as Jean Austin has pointed out, a total condition in which man feels safe.[24] This desire to escape from the unhappy, real life is understandable, but it is an illusory phantasy. Human life entails a lot of pain and unhappiness, although it may have moments of pleasure and happiness. The plain truth is that happiness cannot be procured through scientific knowledge, and that the unhappiness of the neurotic who experiences his life as meaningless cannot be relieved by a faith constructed in a rational manner out of scientific concepts.

VIKTOR E. FRANKL'S ONTOLOGICAL VALUE ETHICS

Fromm's humanistic approach to the problem of neurosis fails because of its deterministic-scientific and hedonistic foundation. We shall now enquire into a psychiatric-ethical approach which is based on an ontological, partly libertarian premise. The author is Viktor E. Frankl.

Frankl's account of human existence 'attempts [an] analysis in the ontological sense, namely an explication, an unfolding of the essence of personal existence'. He postulates a threefold 'dimensional ontology' comprising the somatic, the psychic, and the noetic extensions.[25] The somatic and the psychic areas are taken to be governed by the principle of determinism. Such interpretation is obvious for the somatic field and applies to those psychic disturbances which arise directly from some bodily disturbance. Frankl quotes in particular disorders of the thyroid, the adrenal and the parathyroid glands which according to him can bring about specific neurotic disturbances requiring the administration of specific drugs.

Within the deterministic psychic field, Frankl includes 'the drives' which are, according to him, the drive for pleasure, considered by Freud, and the drive for power, stressed by Adler.

The third extension is the dimension of freedom and values. It is here that man is expected to transcend himself and to find meaning in his life. In this area, we are told, noogenic neuroses arise from conflicts between values and from a lack of fulfilment of spiritual realities. The noogenic treatment consists in logotherapy which 'considers man as a being whose main concern consists in fulfilling a meaning and in actualizing values rather than in the gratification and satsifaction of drives and instincts, in compromising the conflicting claims of id, ego and superego, or in the adaptation and adjustment to society and environment'.[26] (The last alternative refers to the Adlerian view.)

The logotherapist evokes man's will to meaning which may be latent or unconscious. He makes him aware of the hidden *logos* in his existence thus enabling him to fill his existential vacuum which, according to Frankl, is manifest in 'the mass neurosis of the present time', a form of nihilism which is defined as 'the contention that being has no meaning'. The dynamics in the spiritual field are identified as the tension between 'one pole represented by a meaning to be fulfilled and the other pole by the man who *has* to fulfill it'. This tension is considered essential for normal and for neurotic people. The therapist who has diagnosed a noogenic neurosis is thus encouraged to 'increase that load which is brought about by a reorientation toward the meaning of one's life'.[27]

The values are elaborated. They are divided into three types: (a) the creative values which are realized when a task is achieved; (b) the experiential values which are brought about when the Beautiful, the Good or the True are experienced or one single human being is perceived in his uniqueness in a loving relationship; and (c) the attitudinal values which result from 'the very attitude with which we face our destined suffering. . . an achievement of meaning through suffering . . . when the suffering is unavoidable and unescapable'.[28]

Frankl gives many examples which demonstrate how his logotherapy 'attempts to orient and to direct the patient to a concrete, personal meaning'. 'We want,' says Frankl, 'to enable the patient to find his life's meaning. We broaden his field of vision, as it were, so that he may become aware of the full spectrum of his possibilities for personal and concrete meanings and values.'[29]

Men who can see no more possibilities of actualizing 'creative values' are given new hope and strength by being shown the task of helping others, and 'attitudinal values' are evoked when people who suffer from incurable illnesses are presented with the possibilities of enduring suffering as a worthwhile task. Frankl interprets the help which he gives to his patients in terms of his ontological ethics. This interpretation is, however, unconvincing; for the dynamics are confused.

Frankl's spiritual dimension contains a hierarchy of values and an 'ultimate meaning' of a person's life is said to be represented by the 'hierarchically highest value'.[30] One is bound to ask how a collision of values occurs within the hierarchy, what the lower values in the hierarchy and what non-ultimate meanings are. There are no answers to these questions.

The ontological scheme distorts the significance of freedom which is manifest in self-transcendence and in authenticity. According to Frankl, 'only as man withdraws from himself in the sense of releasing self-centred interest and attention will he gain an authentic mode of existence'.[31] The argument is that 'only insofar as a person is capable of ignoring and forgetting himself is he able to recognize anything in and of the world'; the world refers in this context to 'that transcendent sphere of human existence in which man chooses what he will do and what he will be in the midst of an objective world of meanings and values'.[32]

Frankl informs us how patients can enter into this sphere: he advises the use of two techniques, of the 'paradoxical intention' and of 'de-reflexion'. Although these techniques may well be helpful in certain cases, their beneficial effect cannot be explained as the result of a person having exercised his freedom which has gained him access to the 'sphere of meanings and values'.

De-reflexion consists in turning a patient away from himself, from his self-centredness. Frankl gives the following example: a woman was suffering from a fear of choking, which became progressively worse as she observed herself when swallowing. She was given the formula: 'I need not observe the act of swallowing, especially as I do not have to swallow; for it is not me that swallows – it swallows' (what matters is the reliance on the unconscious and unintended automatic reflex).[33]

The paradoxical intention also consists of a command which the patient gives to himself. This technique expects the person to laugh at himself, to be ironical about his fears and his morbid anticipations. Thus he takes the wind out of the sails of his neurotic illness by exaggerating the expected trouble so as to make it ridiculous. For instance, a man who suffered from excessive perspiration of his hands when embarrassed was told to suggest to himself 'I only sweated out a litre before, but now I'm going to pour out at least 10 litres'.[34]

Whereas in de-reflexion the patient is turned away from his fears by the therapist, in the paradoxical intention he must find the strength himself to counteract these fears by being ironical about himself. Through such tricks a person may be freed from very troublesome symptoms, but he does not achieve a meaningful existence, as such an existence is not tantamount to freedom from symptoms of anxiety and complusion.

The sphere of meaning is supposed to be the noetic, spiritual dimension in which the will to meaning is active as an expression of a man's freedom. Frankl holds that 55 per cent of patients and staff in his clinic show 'a more or less marked degree of existential frustration and/or vacuum. More than half of them experienced a loss of the feeling that life is meaningful',[35] but only 14 per cent of patients who are in need of psychotherapy are diagnosed as sufferers from noogenic neuroses. Thus, Frankl concludes, not every neurosis is the result of a conflict affecting conscience or values.[36]

According to Frankl's ontological scheme, sexual neuroses require Freudian scientific treatment to deal with the 'will-to-pleasure' and superiority-complex neuroses need the Adlerian deterministic approach to cope with the 'will-to-power'. Only noogenic neuroses are said to qualify for logotherapy which is based on the 'will-to-meaning'. This account of the neuroses, which follows from the ontological conception, is misleading; for the three wills are wrongly put side by side.[37]

The will-to-meaning is the over-all will; it represents the essence of existential approach.[38] The other two wills represent challenges, which the will-to-meaning has to meet. They are challenges of different kinds and should therefore not be co-ordinated, as in Frankl's theory. The sexual will is the instinctual desire which, while pressing for satisfaction, can bring a person into conflict within his 'spiritual dimension' unless sexual attraction coincides with non-sexual love.

The will to attain status is born out of a feeling of inferiority, as Adler correctly stated. It is a neurotic will and leads to endless conficts within the sphere of values, as it is opposed to the 'loving relationship' between people which Frankl values so greatly. In order to avoid neurotic breakdowns, Adler demands that the will-to-power should be suppressed, whereas Freud insisted that the will-to-[sexual] pleasure should be given more expression.

The existential therapist does not aim either at the suppression or the free expression of these wills, but at their confrontation with the particular person's conscience so that he can come to terms with the conscious and unconscious demands of these potent volitional forces and can achieve a meaningful existence by integrating them within his realm of values.

Frankl's ontological value ethics are no guide to the sufferer from the noogenic neurosis and cannot enable him to gain faith. Although it is customary to distinguish between body, mind, and spirit, this division does not lend itself to a classification of conflicts and to a practice of deterministic and existential psychotherapies.

PERSONALISTIC EXISTENTIAL ETHICS

Freedom of the personal self

The central idea in an ethic which can enable contemporary man to overcome his moral crisis is the personal self, the individual human personality. Such an ethic implies the recognition of values, as they are created and experienced by the self. In the formulation of this philosophy, several pitfalls must be avoided.

(a) The self must not be divorced from the ethical principle, therefore self-actualization must mean the actualization of an ethical self. In his opposition to personalistic ethics, Frankl misinterpreted this basic idea when he asked. 'What would be the result if a man should merely actualize the potentials within himself?' and when, referring to Socrates' admitted criminal tendencies, he replied: 'If he [Socrates] had succeeded in fully developing his potentialities, this great defender of law and justice would also have been a common criminal.' The word 'also' reveals the fault of Frankl's argument. Socrates could not have developed into a common criminal and into a genuine great defender of law and justice. The self which he realized was the moral self.[39]

(b) A further source of confusion arises from a general, meta-physical-ontological interpretation of self-realization which presumes that the self, left to itself, realizes itself. Such a theory is meaningless to the sufferers from the noogenic neuroses; they need a philosophy which calls for an effort of transcending themselves to gain personal freedom.

(c) There is the danger from deterministic psychology. This science operates with the self concept and postulates that the self is knowable as a measurable, fixed entity. It requires such a self concept for the formulation of valid psychological laws. Personalistic ethics postulates the freedom of the self and thus does not accept the scientific, deterministic framework of the psychologist.[40]

The idea of the free self which is basic to the argument in this book has been clarified by Karl Jaspers. He has pointed out that 'to scientific objective cognition of the world there is no such thing as freedom. Hence freedom cannot be visualized in a defined concept'. Jaspers offers an alternative to the clarity of unambiguous cognition, and we shall follow him. He says: 'However, that which I cannot know objectively, I can nevertheless become familiar with by thinking, can bring to conceptual actuality in the movement of thought.' But he adds this warning '. . .it is inevitable that it will contain a maze of misconceptions'.[41]

This movement of thought, reflection, is itself one of the manifestations of personal freedom and the conceptual actuality is an achievement of the striving for freedom. The person who practices his freedom of reflecting on his own lack of freedom, becomes aware of his situation. He may be rewarded; his exercise of freedom may, in Jaspers' words, yield 'a release from the obscure bondage of the undifferentiated, from the given thus-ness of the self (Sosein), from the power of uncritically accepted symbols and from the absolute reality of the objective world'. Such a person may agree with Jaspers: 'It is a relief that at last I know what up to then I have only felt. If I know what happens to me, I have taken the first step to freedom in contrast to being blindly overpowered.'[42]

Jaspers has described several facets of awareness, each of which involves an 'outward' and an 'inward' perception. They are all achievements of personal freedom and they consist of (1) the self's awareness of its environment and of the impression it makes on others; (2) the self's awareness of a situation in which it has been placed and this situation's effect on the self, taking into account personal disposition, sensitivity and strength of coping; and (3) the self's awareness of the social milieu with regard to its own social obligations and to its own social importance to others. As Jaspers remarks, in all these respects, the self perceives its particular individuality and at the same time its value. Such affirmation of selfhood is experienced as 'meaningful connections'.[43]

Personalistic ethics, which are based on the affirmation of a potentially free self, are existential in the sense in which P. Foulquié has defined this term: 'To exist is to take leave of what one is (ex) in order to establish oneself (sistere) on the level which formerly was only possible.'[44]

Modern man in his ethical crisis can save himself if he adopts the philosophy of personal existential ethics. Dissatisfied with his state of existence, he must assert his self's freedom and establish his existence on a new level. In his efforts, he must aim at authenticity and must transcend his personal self.

Authenticity and transcendence

Existential writers do not agree on the meaning of the terms authenticity and transcendence. Rollo May holds that a man can reach authenticity by going through different stages of consciousness. He lists the following phases: (1) the innocence of the infant before a conscious self has arisen; (2) the rebellion of the small child and of the adolsecent who fights for his freedom; (3) 'the ordinary consciousness of self', which is gained when 'a person can to some extent see his errors, make some allowance for his prejudices, use his guilt feelings and anxiety as experiences to learn from, and make his decisions with some responsibility'. May adds to this description the remark: 'This is what most people mean when they speak of a healthy state of personality.'[45]

We are concerned with those who have not achieved this healthy state, who are in need of a new existence. We therefore turn to (4) transcendence. Unfortunately, not much hope is offered here to all those whose existence is inauthentic and who suffer from the emptiness of their lives.

The fourth stage, we are told, is extraordinary and 'most individuals experience it only rarely'. It is reached when we get sudden insights, in dreams or 'at moments of reverie'. These are moments of clarity, provided by the rise of knowledge from the subconscious, also moments of creativity, whether of the scientific or religious or artistic kind. These are moments of objective truth, of 'self-surpassing consciousness'. The stage is thus called the 'creative consciousness of self'.[46]

Persons in this rare state are said to be in ecstasy, to stand outside themselves, to experience the world from a perspective outside the limited usual viewpoint, and not to be suffering from the clouded subjectivity of the ordinary person. According to May, people can reach this state only very occasionally, as it is mainly for the saint and for the great creative figure.[47]

Rollo May, who is a prominent existentialist and therapist, does not relate in his *Man's Search for Himself* his theory to his practice. Another well-known existential author and therapist, J. F. T. Bugental, has applied his views on authenticity and transcendence to his psychotherapy.

Bugental's book is entitled *The Search for Authenticity* and its sub-title is *An Existential-Analytic Approach to Psychotherapy.* To him, authenticity is the central concern of psychotherapy and he gives the following definition of the authentic person: 'A person is authentic in that degree to which his being in the world is unqualifiedly in accord with the givenness of his own nature and of the world. . . Authenticity is the term I will use to characterize both an hypothesized ultimate state of at-oneness with the cosmos and the immense continuum leading toward that ultimate ideal.'[48]

Since, according to Bugental, 'neurosis consists in the denial or distortion of authenticity', psychotherapy is interpreted as the medium which enables the patient to discard 'some of the constrictions he has put on himself-and-his-world sufficiently to recognize their limiting and hurtful effects', thus increasing his authenticity.[49]

Bugental's treatment is divided into phases: the first phase is analytic, in it the patient is made aware of himself and his inner world, social constraints are dissolved and thoughts, impulses and feelings are explored.[50]

The second phase is called ontogogy, it is 'concerned with aiding a person to actualize or make real more of his potential once the grosser handicapping effects of his emotional disruption have been overcome'.[51]

Numerous examples are quoted as illustrations of the second phase. As in the first place, awareness plays a prominent part. The difference appears to be that the resistance to awareness is dealt with in the first phase, whereas in the second phase the patient has gained awareness of the self-fragmentation which bars him from becoming authentic.

The third phase represents the state of transcendence, 'an hypothetized point of full authenticity of being in which the person would emerge into oneness with the All. There is no non-mystical language really available for describing this concept. By its very nature it partakes of mystery or mysticism – it is unknown to our usual understanding. Transcendence implies the complete confronting and incorporating of existential anxiety in all its forms. . . Transcendence is complete awareness and full feelingful assent'.[52]

'Ontological freedom is an estate to be aspired to but seldom achieved.' Bugental postulates different levels of this state.[53] The highest level is reached when 'the boundary between I and world is experienced as fluid and changing with one's awareness and experience. The Me or Self is recognized for what it is, a scrapbook of the past, interesting, personal, but static and not binding upon the liberated I that lives in this minute'.[54]

The author seems himself worried about the implications of his assumptions, for he says of this truly emancipated person that he would be 'a very different sort of person than most of us, somewhat difficult for us to communicate with and rather frightening to know'. The comforting thought is that in fact such people do not exist, although this 'newer celebration of our being' may be realized in the future.[55] This hope is, however, no consolation to all the neurotic people who also fail to fulfil Rollo May's conditions of supreme creativity and saintliness. A more practical approach to the attainment of transcendence and authenticity must be found, it must be available to the millions of people who have lost faith and who suffer from the general neurosis of our time.

Personalistic existential ethics provides an answer to man's urgent needs. Although it affirms the right of the person, it goes beyond the postulate of personal self-hood. This going beyond is transcendence. Faith refers to transcendence, to the possibilities of freedom. As Karl Jaspers has pointed out, 'it is only through freedom that I become certain of transcendence'.[56] Transcendence, thus understood, is not reserved for saints or mystics. It is the prerogative of the ordinary person, including the neurotic.

Jaspers shows how the finite person depends for his authenticity on transcendence: 'he must be given to himself over and over again, if he is not to lose himself'.[57] The proof that transcendence is the light by which all – religious and non-religious men – live, lies in the fact that without it, the essential tasks of life cannot be carried out. As Jaspers put it, 'if man maintains his inner integrity in the face of fate and even death, he cannot do so by himself alone. What helps him here is of a different kind than any help in the world. Transcendent help reveals itself to him solely in the fact that he can be himself. That he can stand by himself, he owes to an intangible hand, extended to him from transcendence, a hand whose presence he can feel only in his freedom'.[58] He who finds life empty and senseless, who suffers from the noogenic neurosis, can save himself by the discovery of transcendence.

Transcendence is not just an absolute, theoretical principle, a concept in a philosophical system. It is experienced as the 'basic trait' in human consciousness in man's inner world.[59] An account of existential ethics must clarify the relationship of freedom to this inner world of experience.

Freedom in relation to the inner world

A systematic approach to the inner world of experience was earlier described as 'phenomenological psychiatry'. Wilhelm Dilthey's distinction between intuitive understanding of the mind and conceptual psychological knowledge was quoted above and phenomenological psychiatry was criticized for its deterministic framework which considers that patients are confined to the worlds of their mental and emotional illnesses.

In contrast to such denial of freedom, existential ethics conceives the inner worlds as being open, presenting the self with potentialities of new experiences. The freedom of experience must, however, not be separated from the ethical freedom, but must be subordinated under it. Existential ethics accepts the freedom of experience as a means of gaining a greater measure of authenticity. In order to clarify the significance of phenomenology for existential ethics, we have to enquire into the existential application of Edmund Husserl's phenomenology.

Husserl took the data of consciousness as his starting point to obtain an *a priori* knowledge of Being, an insight into essences. We are not concerned with this 'eidetic science', but with the individual's subjective world and his freedom in this world.

Husserl called the relationship between the self and his experience intentional, by which he meant that data of consciousness cannot be separated from the self, but that the self sends out a 'shaft of attention' which terminates in the object of consciousness.[60] There is no empty consciousness, only consciousness with contents which are the experiences and 'the bearers of the specific quality of intentionality' such as colour, touch, sound, pleasure, pain, and a feeling of animation.[61]

Whereas for Husserl the act of intentionality was the basis for the eidetic science and whereas consciousness to him referred to a universal human attribute, we are concerned with the individual person's consciousness. By accepting the notion of intentionality, of activity on the part of the self, we accept not only the interrelatedness of the subject and his world, but also the notion of freedom which is entailed in the act of intentionality. Thus we do not conceive the realm of experience as something passive and unalterable, but, on the contrary, as something which the individual self has brought about consciously or unconsciously and which he has the freedom to change.[62]

For an explanation of experience, we have to assume unconscious activity of the self. Husserl postulated that the shaft of attention stood out in full clearness, but he made also allowance for 'a fringe of background inattention showing relative differences of clearness and obscurity', as well as for 'emphasis and lack of relief'.[63] Through making the self aware of this background, we bring obscure areas into the full light of attention and become free to change the world of our experience.

The constitution of our inner world (which phenomenological psychiatry systematizes by references to mental illnesses) is not accidental. It is not the result of any natural, deterministic forces, but of our attitudes, desires, and evaluations which we have some freedom to change.

Intentionality is preconscious, it precedes the stage at which we can formulate our thoughts and knowledge of our world. M. Merleau-Ponty, quoting Husserl, called this important activity operative intentionality, and characterized it as 'that which produces the natural and antepredicative unity of the world and of our life, being apparent in our desires, our evaluations and in the landscape we see, more clearly than in objective knowledge, and furnishing the text which our knowledge tries to translate into precise language'.[64] By becoming aware of this operative intentionality, man becomes free to alter its product to some extent. By realizing his freedom towards his inner world, he realizes his freedom also in relation to his outer world.

Freedom in relation to the outer world

In Husserl's philosophy, the outer world is 'put into brackets', that is, it is excluded from the phenomenological standpoint. Reality as outside reality is not considered, as Husserl was concerned only with the consciousness of the 'real' world and not with reality as such.

The person who is not intent to gain absolute knowledge, but who is intent to live in the world, does not confine himself to Husserl's phenomenological point of view. He recognizes his responsibilities in the world around him. He can meet them only if he moves from the inner to the outer world.

Martin Buber has clarified the ways in which man can approach the outer world. Two attitudes are available to him: first the 'I-It' posture, a detached relationship to objects which he handles, observes, and knows 'without any feeling for their exclusiveness'.[65] In this frame of mind, we perceive events as set in time and space. Many creative activities, including scientific work, are carried out on this objective basis. Causality reigns in the world of the It, and 'without It man cannot live'.

Buber goes on to say, 'But he who lives with It alone is not a man'.[66] Man is in need of the world of the Thou. 'Through the *Thou* a man becomes *I*',[67] becomes confirmed in his selfhood by another self in the I-Thou relationship. Although the Thou appears in space and in time, the I-Thou relationship is lived independently of the space-time co-ordinates.[68] Man becomes conscious of his transcendence in the I-Thou relationship, in which he is assured of his freedom.

This freedom is lost if a person does not relate himself to another person, in Buber's language if the 'inborn *Thou*' does not meet a *Thou* in the outer world. In such a case, he says, 'the inborn Thou. . . strikes inwards. It develops on the unnatural, impossible object of the *I*, that is, it develops where there is no place at all for it to develop.'[69]

An object like a tree or an animal can speak to man as a Thou, but the I-Thou relationship is mostly between man and man. Alas, it does not last, it deteriorates into an I-It relationship, in which man makes use of the other as an object. Buber points out, 'it is the exalted melancholy of our fate that every *Thou* in our world must become an *It*'.[70] It is up to the persons concerned to re-build the I-Thou relationship and never to take each other for granted.

The I-Thou relationship requires two whole people to conduct the genuine dialogue in which 'each should regard his partner as the very one he is',[71] accepting him and confirming him as a partner.

Buber like Jaspers complains that the present age is not conducive to the development of I-Thou relationships. The 'mystery' of the inter-human life is destroyed by the scientific-analytical attitude which objectifies the psyche.

Freedom of decision

Apart from communicating with a fellow human being, man communicates with himself so that he can arrive at decisions and choices which manifest his freedom, but which also require guidance from principles and norms.

He who has lost faith in God must make his own norms. 'Man, therefore, advances in life as in a starless night along a road bordered with precipices. . . Day will not come. . . life goes on without him, and not to make a choice is to leave the decision to blind chance.'[72]

Existential philosophers, such as Sartre, Jaspers, and Heidegger all agree that 'only the man who chooses freely to be himself, who makes himself, who is his own work, can truly be said to exist'.[73] By making the choice, by deciding either/or, man confers authenticity upon himself and dares to make the leap of faith of which Kierkegaard spoke. A person becomes certain of his transcendence in the absoluteness of his decisions.

Modern man has recognized his image in the characters created by Sartre, in people who do not find the courage to make decisions and thus to exercise the freedom of their existence. This is the neurotic image.

In *Nausea,* the Self-Taught man, asked by the waitress to choose his dessert, turns white, unable to answer.[74] Matthieu, the hero in the novel *The Roads to Freedom,* finishes his life in a hopeless battle against the invading German Army, deploring his life-long indecisiveness: 'Each of his shots avenged some ancient scruple. One for Lola whom I dared not rob; one for Marcelle whom I ought to have left in the lurch; one for Odette whom I didn't want to kiss. This for the books I never dared to write, this for the journeys I never made, this for everybody in general whom I wanted to hate and tried to understand. . . He fired. He was cleansed. He was all-powerful. He was free.'[75]

Personalistic existential ethics realizes that life offers man choices of opposite possibilities; we therefore lose what we reject and gain what we choose. As Jaspers has put it, 'we must always accept the opposite, risk it, let it become a thorn of distress and include it as a factor in all our movements. Anything that merely is without an opposite means fixation, loss of all otherness and soon an end to all that has already become lifelessly fixated. But when we expose ourselves to the reciprocal dialectic movement and risk, life expands its meaning'.[76] He who shrinks from taking the risk of a decision is guilty before his conscience.

Freedom of conscience

The notion of conscience needs clarification. A. Duncan-Jones has surveyed the different meanings which have been attached to this term.[77] He had distinguished three interpretations: conscience conceived (1) as a rational power in a moral sense, (2) as a mode of moral perception and (3) as moral emotion. The last interpretation does not imply that the voice of conscience is reliable, whereas the first two involve such a claim. Reason is credited with the ability to apprehend truth and the moral sense theory, likening conscience to such abilities as seeing and hearing, postulates that man has a moral sense which tells him what he ought to do (or not to do) in individual situations. Such a theory assumes that conscience is as trustworthy as eyesight and hearing.

In his paper Duncan-Jones has given two reasons why modern people have lost faith in the reliability of conscience: (1) anthropologists have shown – or seem to have shown – that there is almost endless diversity among the moral codes and rules which prevail in different societies: and that most individuals adopt as a matter of course the morality which prevails at the place and time at which they grew up and (2) certain psychologists hold that conscience is formed under the influence of the family and is thus a product of the home environment.[78]

Duncan-Jones has agreed with the anthropological and psychological sceptical views but, nevertheless, holds that the individual person has the freedom to reflect upon his conduct and is not forced to accept a moral code from society or his family. In spite of such acknowledgement, this conventional moral philosopher, tied to the notion of theoretical consistency, cannot justify the assumption of conscience. To him this faculty would have to be omniscient, never leaving its bearer in any doubt as to the correct choice in a perplexing moral situation; this condition cannot be fulfilled.

Personalistic existential ethics does not insist on the infallibility of conscience. Far from considering the possibility of an insoluble moral conclict as an invalidation, it sees in such a crisis a confirmation of conscience. Because of inevitable ethical dilemmas, man has to bear guilt in such situations, no matter what decision he might make.

Numerous examples of irreconcilable duties can be quoted. Albert Schweitzer provided such an illustration when he discussed the implications of vivisection. Man violates animal life in order to save human life.[79]

In his *Existentialism and Humanism,* Jean-Paul Sartre asked: should a young Frenchman perform his duty towards his country during the German occupation as a soldier in the resistance movement or should he stay with his elderly mother who needs his support? Sartre was right when he concluded that there is no golden rule of morality which would enable the young man to answer the question correctly, and that he cannot gain perfect peace of mind whichever alternative he chooses.[80]

Sartre touched upon the human problem of ordinary people even more directly in his comments on the following story: Maggi Tulliver, a character in *The Mill on the Floss* is passionately in love with Stephen, but gives him up, as he is engaged to another woman. This duty to respect the engagement is contradicted by the fact that the rival is an insignificant person, incapable of passion which – according to Stendhal, quoted by Sartre – takes preference over the banality of love which awaits Stephen in his marriage with 'the little goose'. Maggie feels the 'right' of her passion but decides in favour of the ethic which takes the engagement as an absolute bar to exercising this right.[81]

As Schweitzer has pointed out, society has no claim to lay down rules of ethics for the individual. 'The collapse of civilization has come about through ethics being left to society. . . A renewal. . . is possible only if ethics become once more the concern of thinking human beings, and if individuals seek to assert themselves in society as ethical personalities.'[82] Thus conscience is personal.

He who evades his personal duty is guilty. His consicence tells him when he fails to make the right use of his potentialities, when he wastes his life. Guilt also occurs when man does not fulfil his duties towards others. Martin Buber defined existential guilt as 'guilt that a person has taken on himself as a person and in a personal situation', and that guilt 'occurs when someone injures an order of the human world whose foundations he knows and recognizes as those of his own existence and of all common human existence'.[83]

Conscience can be unconscious, but it can be elevated[84] into consciousness or can be suppressed. The man who hears the call of conscience, who is conscious of his tasks in life, finds life meaningful and becomes aware of the road to authenticity. The person who is not aware of conscience is apt to find life meaningless, as he has no means of orientating himself. The sufferers from the noogenic neurosis belong to the last group.

Limitations of personal freedom

The sufferers from the noogenic neurosis are sick people and their sickness limits their ability to hear the voice of conscience and to carry out its command. What man can face and what he can do about it depends to some extent on what he is, on his capacity for moral discernment, and his moral fibre. In an ethic which is medically orientated freedom is restricted.

The acknowledgement of the limitations of freedom does not imply the acceptance of determinism as the overall principle and does not mean the abolition of personalistic existential ethics. Freedom is safeguarded in two respects.

Firstly, from the subjective-experiential point of view: a person is left with the possibility of *facing* his limitations, of coming to terms with them, which means that he can exercise his freedom within the bondage of his restrictions. Secondly, from an objective point of view: the limitations may be temporary, the ethical force may break through the barrier of sickness.

The assessment of a person's moral capacity is the outcome of scientific-deterministic studies, which are concerned with the genetic constitution, with historical-cultural factors and with biological (especially cerebral) conditions. The uncertainty with regard to the correct forecast of the effects of these scientifically knowable factors is, however, not interpreted as being the result of unpredictable variations in the genetic, historical-social, or biological patterns. The uncertainty is not subject to the causality of any of the sciences, it does not belong to the realm of science which is governed by the presupposition of determinism. The uncertainty belongs to the realm of personal ethics which admits that a person's moral strength varies, and that the freedom of existence is not a force which, like the force which physicists study, can be measured and expected to follow a determinable course.

The limitations of freedom violate only the theoretical consistency, not the practical value of the personalistic existential philosophy. Just as in the case of conscience, certainty was sacrificed to the possibility of doubt, so in the case of the freedom of existence, unbreakable strength gives way to moral frailty. Such a solution may be less satisfying philosophically than Kant's formulation according to which man belongs to two realms, the sphere of scientific phenomena and the domain of spiritual noumena, but it has the advantage of being more adaptable to human needs.

The limitation of freedom varies from one person to the next and also at different times in the same person's life. The assessment of restrictions and potentialities and the ways of coming to terms with lack of freedom will be discussed in the next chapter which deals with the therapeutic applications of personalistic existential ethics.

Before enquiring into the psychopathology which arises from the unavoidable limitations of freedom, we must counter those influences which sabotage human existence. Freedom is threatened by presumptions made by scientists and philosophers who have overstepped the boundaries of legitimate determinism. We shall answer the scientists first.

4

Intensification of Neurosis Through Scientific and Philosophical Presumptions

PRESUMPTIONS OF SCIENTISM

Scientists, who are by profession determinists, violate personal freedom if they interpret the human mind in a deterministic way. As neurosis was shown to be a moral phenomenon and as its treatment must be based on personalistic ethics which affirms the freedom of existence, these scientists intensify neurotic suffering and tend to prevent the adoption of the right therapeutic measures. Because of the general respect for scientific knowledge, people are liable to agree to these unwarranted claims and to their implications. In defence of the sufferers from noogenic neurosis, we must expose the fallacy of their presumptions and must repudiate the explanation of the personality in terms of physical, biological, psychological, evolutionary, and historical deterministic theories. As such a use of science is in fact an abuse, it can be called a scientism, a term which has been coined to denote a faulty scientific methodology. We shall start with the scientism of physics, with physicalism.

Physicalism

To W. Card 'the data which a sick patient presented were the ultimate atomic facts of the manifestations of disease'.[1] The underlying conception is physicalistic, a faulty application of mathematical physics to the practice of medicine. It assumes that the suffering of sick people can be reduced to identical, ultimate data which can be calculated by the computer. The consequences of this reduction are evident in the title of Card's lecture, 'Hippocratic Era Ending. . .' which, as the lecturer said himself, has survived for over two thousand years as 'the era of traditional medicine'.[2]

Traditional Hippocratic medicine is based on the personal relationship between doctor and patient which entails the ethical special I-Thou quality that the patient needs in order to bear his disease and to find the courage to strive for health. To Card, the doctor's task is entirely related to the computer; 'to elicit clinical signs and symptoms', the doctor's personality is unnecessary, which is evident from the lecturer's plan 'to test the performance of an intelligent computer-aided nurse against a consultant'.[3]

A. R. Feinstein goes even further in his enthusiasm for computers than W. Card. He demands that computers should be used 'for patient, not disease'. He holds that computers can 'rehumanize clinical medicine' by having been programmed with 'all the data – information about the patient as well as the disease'.[4]

Feinstein's programme cannot be realized, for the information about the patient, considered as a human being and not as a bearer of a classifiable disease, lies outside the realm of the computer, since it refers to his uniqueness.

Apart from data reduction, physicalism encroaches upon the person's freedom through identifying the mind with physical matter (which is knowable by physics). Some scientists usurp the mind via the body, in particular via the brain. A representative of this school is J. Z. Young whose first aim is 'to bridge the gap between biology and engineering'.[5] He does not only compare biological structures such as the brain with physical structures such as homeostats (which include computers), but, in spite of the dissimilarity between brains and comouters (which he admits) decides to speak of the brain in the language of the computer.[6] He thus describes the nervous system in engineering terms.[7]

After equating living matter with dead matter, Young treats the mind as being equivalent to the brain and to the computer, which means that to him, the mind is also no different from matter. Memory for instance is to Young the physical representation of the world in which an animal or a man lives, and the representation is stored in certain cells in the brain, the dendritic cells.[8] (The brain has not only access to the individual memory, but also to the hereditary memory, using a pre-established code or alphabet.[9]) This physicalistic interpretation of memory eliminates the creative activities of the individual human mind; it is not a theoretical framework which serves the elucidation of a particular scientific problem – the legitimate use of analogues and models in science – but it presumes to make metaphysical, irrefutable statements about human nature.

If, according to Young, 'calculating machines and brains both think',[10] the question can seriously be discussed whether there is any difference between people and robots.[11]

To the inspired machine-theorist the machine has a mind and is conscious of concepts, as it could not think otherwise. In his article entitled 'Could A Machine Perceive?' Alan Gauld shows that the machine theorist uses a machine-table which can be embodied in a digital computer and that a 'machine specified by this table would simulate some parts of the real Jones's behaviour quite closely',[12] but that a human mind does not work just in terms of input and output. Although machines can play games as human beings can, machines are ignorant of such notions as rule, criterion, success, skill, and luck.[13]

Gauld's refutation is not radical. It is not directed against the basic physicalistic standpoint and it misses the vital difference between man and a product of his own inventiveness.

Some leaders of the medical profession are aware of the danger from physicalism. Lord Platt is one of them. He chose for his Harveian Oration the title 'Medical Science: Master or Servant?' Lord Platt objects to the view which reduces man to 'a chemical engine' and stresses as man's true attributes 'the endless variety of the interplay of human personality, intellect, emotion and motivation'.[14] He warns against the neglect of the patient which follows from physicalism in medicine.

Well-known authorities on the science of physics have intensified man's moral crisis by their adoption of physicalism. An example was P. W. Bridgman. In his *The Way Things Are,* this winner of a Nobel Prize stated that 'there is nothing inconsistent in supposing that the various modes of subconscious activity to which the psychoanalyst gives special names such as "id" or "superego" correspond to recognizable patterns in the atomic activity of the brain'.[15] This physicalistic interpretation is fallacious as it relates the dynamics of the psyche to those of the physical constituents of the body, thereby ignoring the fundamental differences between these two realms!

Physicalism is not only proclaimed by the representatives of rigorous sciences, it is also announced by influential popular authors and thus reaches the common man. Marshall McLuhan is such a writer.

McLuhan identifies the central nervous system with an 'electrical network that coordinates the various media of our senses'.[16] This definition is called a 'physiological' statement. Such a sentence is misleading in two respects: firstly, the central nervous system is not an electrical network, only a physicalist reduces a living structure to a dead thing; and secondly, this physicalistically converted object would not obey the laws of physiology, but the laws of physics. The truth is that technology has changed man's perception of the world, has influenced human relations, and has thus affected the human mind deeply. It has certainly provided new opportunities to man, as McLuhan has pointed out. For instance, modern man can gain information on all sorts of subjects through television, but electricity is not sheer information, as McLuhan asserts,[17] nor is information electricity. McLuhan called his book *Understanding Media*. . . but he does not understand media, as the media which are the fruits of technology are interpreted biologically, and as the science of technology itself is described as 'an extension of his [man's] physical body',[18] which is another physicalistic statement, making a product of the mind, a science, into a physical object.

The serious problem which confronts man is whether he is the master or servant of his own intentions. Freedom, however, is not lost if, through proper understanding, through awareness of the technological situation, man can discover new possibilities for the development of himself. The doctrine of physicalism tends to confuse the human mind and to prevent self-liberation.

Biologism

Physicalism reduces the person to a physical object, biologism to a biological object. The biologistic error stems from the faulty conception of the relationship between body and mind which, we found, misguides the biological psychiatrist. Although biological (neurological) knowledge is relevant for the connections between brain and mind, it does not provide knowledge of the mind. By imposing its deterministic framework biologism, like physicalism, is corruptive, denying human freedom. A paper by William Sargant, entitled 'The Physiology of Faith',[19] illustrates the biologistic error.

As in Young's physicalism, the brain is identified with a computer. To this physicalistic scientism Sargant adds the biologistic scientism, as computing is made into a neurophysiological event. The distinction between critical and uncritical computing is basic to the 'physiology of faith'. The former is said to lead to scientifically established faith, the latter to faith which as yet rests on no sure foundation.[20] The second type of faith, according to Sargant, is the result of cerebral overstimulation (as, for instance, produced by the beating of drums in primitive societies) or of abnormal brain inhibition (as in mystical contemplation). Two types of uncritical faith are cited: faith in God and in psycho-analysis. No evidence of over- or under-stimulation responsible for the emergence of psycho-analytic faith is offered.

To those who use critical non-computer judgement Sargant's account suffers from the following fallacies.

(1) By introducing critical judgement, a mind is in fact postulated. Although such a mind depends on a brain, the mind and not the brain acts critically (or uncritically). Nerve cells cannot be said to have

judgement. Logical thinking cannot be derived from physiological data, although an intact physiological cerebral apparatus is essential for intellectual performance.[21]

(2) By postulating an identical cerebral physiological foundation for all mental phenomena, Sargant is led to the use of the same term to denote forms of human endeavour which are utterly different: religious faith is a transcendental belief which lies outside the boundaries of rationality. It is therefore by its nature uncritical. Scientific faith is not a faith at all; it is the application of the method of science which consists in the formulation of a refutable theory and in testing its validity by observation. This method is rational and critical. Psycho-analytic faith is not a faith either, but a metaphysical doctrine which is irrefutable and from which the functioning of the mind is deduced. Its method is uncritical to the extent to which it is non-scientific, but the argument from the metaphysical premise is conducted rationally.

Sargant's brain physiology, which is meant to explain the three types of faith, is at fault: normal cerebral functioning must be accepted for the scientist, for the Freudian, and for the majority of religious people. It must be admitted, however, that some religious people use psychedelic drugs, exciting movements of the body, stimulating music or bodily isolation, all of which cause alterations in cerebral conditions which may heighten their religious experiences.

Sargant's quotations of Pavlov's experiments on dogs are particularly inappropriate in this context: 'Very strong dogs, who could not be broken down by the conflict situations and excitement artificially created for them, might only break after they had later been physically debilitated, or had their metabolism altered in other ways and then the same disturbing stimuli reapplied. Prolonged fasting, or gastrointestinal upset, a severe fever, or interference with glandular functions, such as by castration, are some of the most effective methods Pavlov found for getting at and altering the behaviour of his strongest and previously most stable dogs.' Whatever happened in the case of these experimental animals, Sargant is wrong in continuing, 'It has been proved to be just the same in man',[22] the same when religious faith is induced.

The physiological changes which Pavlov produced in his dogs made them unstable and better objects for abnormal conditioning. But spiritual experiences and Freudian psychotherapy have nothing to do with animal Pavlovian conditioning. The 'physiology of faith' is logically absurd and morally corruptive.

Biologistically minded psychiatrists do not only suffer and spread confusion with regard to religious values, they also get entangled in contradictions in their own fields, in the study and treatment of emotional illness. An example is W. Malcolm Millar, a professor of mental health.

Millar has lent his strength to the revaluation of a mental condition, hysteria. He deplores the fact that hysterical patients of today are not given the benefits of modern neuropsychiatric knowledge, and he discovers much confusion in the minds of his colleagues. He therefore sets out to clarify the matter. While he cannot agree with current complex psychiatric views, he decides to arrive at a 'simple notion of hysteria', making use of 'accepted scientific standards of reliable and consistent observation and accurate, agreed definition'. Millar describes hysteria as an event, as a state of mind and concludes by eliminating the whole field of psychosomatics: 'In so far as the condition affects bodily functioning it must follow that hysteria is a disorder of the central nervous system.' He chides those who cannot accept such a conclusion: 'There remain some who still hold to peripheral theory – that the particular organ itself is affected.' Millar does not reveal who these people are, but refers to the past by saying: 'This is a relic of the theory of the wandering womb first put forward lightheartedly by Plato.' He then deals sternly with those who hold a psychological theory: 'Likewise there are some who hold to an exclusively psychological theory.' He himself holds exclusively to an organic-biological theory, saying that the psychological theory is nonsensical, 'for we are manifestly concerned with the physical and the tangible'.[23] The rest of the paper does not help in the simplification of the problem, as the author goes into details of the 'personality structure' of the hysterical personality, which he somehow links with a disturbance of the 'autonomous systems', the 'un-integration' which is defined as 'the simple and understandable basis for the hysterical state'.[24]

The confusion of biologism from which Millar's paper suffers becomes obvious in his own application of the neurophysiological theory in an example of a patient who suffered from a hysterical condition; he was a new widower who on the occasion of his wife's funeral was found 'to the horror of everyone, having intercourse with the maid' and who replied to the question "what are you doing?": "How do I know? I'm out of my mind with grief."'[25]

The event of the widower's intercourse cannot be satisfactorily explained on a neurophysiological basis as an 'unintegrated state' of his nervous system, it can only be explained as a state of his mind. Although psychological-deterministic elements, sexual desire, weakness of the ego, and the complex situation of the funeral play important parts, they do not invalidate the moral implications of the event. Millar refers to the deterministic psychological mechanisms in hysteria: identification, dissociation, displacement, conversion, and dramatization. The widower's mind is dissociated. Only a personal analysis could reveal to what extent the other mechanisms contributed to his lapse, but none of them are 'an activation of any of the systems of the Central Nervous System'.[26]

Millar's biologism thus misrepresents the situation in which the hysterical patient finds himself; it denies him the genuineness of his emotional life and reduces him to a neural automaton. Biologism also distorts human relationships. This scientistic error is evident in the writings of Harry Stack Sullivan.

As Leslie H. Farber has pointed out, Sullivan held that 'subjective relations could be studied from the objective viewpoints of a scientist – moreover, of a physical scientist – and that experience could be adequately described in the terminology of the sciences'.[27] As a result of this mistaken belief we find the ethical personal world of the I-Thou reduced to the deterministic, impersonal I-It world of physiological-instinctual processes. We also find spatial and temporal factors to take up a primary causal role instead of providing merely the background for the endeavours of the participants in the human communication.

The love relationship between mother and child provides a good example for demonstrating this scientistic corruption. There is of course a temporal development in this relationship, the child goes through stages of maturing and the mother also changes with regard to her own feelings; but this temporal aspect is in no way primary, and the communication of mutual love does not depend on the stage of development in mother and child, although the expression of love varies at different times.

In Sullivan's book *The Interpersonal Theory of Psychiatry*, the temporal 'developmental epochs' are taken as basic for the understanding of the relationship between mother and child, together with the child's physiological, spatial bodily functions. These objective It factors displace the Thou element which is obviously the essential matter in the relationship. Love itself loses its spontaneous, primary status and is deduced from tensions which 'effect the biological disequilibrium' of the child's being. These tensions are said to be 'primarily appertaining to his [the child's] communal existence with the physicochemical universe'.[28]

An example shows what happens to a mother's love under such scientistic treatment. Sullivan discusses the role which the anal zone plays in the interpersonal relations between mother and child: 'The functional activity centering in the anal zone often becomes involved in the manifestations of infantile anxiety, especially when the [mother] is made anxious by these details of her mothering function'.[29]

It is absurd to make the anal (or any other bodily) zone the cause of anxiety, as the cause lies in the mind which associates prudish ideas with certain parts of the body. Biologism misleads people and tends to prevent them from dealing with their neurotic disturbances in the correct manner.

Psychologism

While biologism denies the existence of the psyche, psychologism accounts for it in terms of psychological determinism. The examination of psychological psychiatry revealed the failure of the scientific approach to the mind, as is evident from Gordon W. Allport's cited admission of the irreconcilable claims of different personality theories.[30] We shall now investigate the significance of this faulty deterministic framework for the appreciation of the free person and shall emphasize first the abuse of deterministic mental mechanisms.

Mechanistic psychologism

The confusion which results from the introduction of mechanistic, scientific concepts into the conception of a whole personality is illustrated by a paper in which Erick H. Erikson discusses the role of identity in a positive and negative sense. A negative identity is a means of fixing elements within us which we dislike, namely 'what we know or fear or are told we are but try not to be or not to see; and what we consequently see in exaggeration in others'.[31]

In the same paper, Erikson shows how the process of identity can lead to hatred among people, but he also shows that a person can refuse to accept negative identity. Erikson's example of such a man is Gandhi.

Gandhi did indeed choose his own identity, which he asserted in his struggle for India's independence. Therefore he did not succumb to the mechanisms of the mind. He exercised his freedom. Gandhi identified himself with non-violence and he trusted his adversaries that they would respond to this image. Erikson, however, makes this response which showed Gandhi's courage, a moral quality, into an automatic instinct-like behaviour; for he finds a parallel in the behaviour of stags, which, when fighting do not exploit the opportunity of piercing an unprotected flank of a rival with an antler. The stags have an 'autonomous instinct' according to Lorenz and their fight is governed by ritual. They are thus not free. But Gandhi risked the hostile response from the people whom he trusted, and his trust had nothing in common with the 'trust' of the stag. Gandhi was not led by something which has a parallel in animal instincts, nor was his identification with the idea of non-violence automatic.

The interpretation of human motivation, of responsible and daring action in psychologistic-mechanistic terms is corruptive; and so is the interpretation of conscience in terms of psychological mechanisms.

The super-ego

The mechanisms of introjection and projection are involved in the dynamics of the super-ego which to a Freudian stands for conscience. The personal super-ego is said to be composed of internalized parental prohibitions, and these introjected objects can be projected, for instance in the shape of policemen or bogeymen. Identification plays a vital role: the child identifies himself with his parents and with their prohibitions.

Freud has opened our eyes to the hidden influence which parents play in the lives of their children. He has demonstrated the power of unconscious mechanisms.

We must admit that we do not only depend on 'internalized' parental views but also on the views of the community in which we live. Thus, apart from acknowledging the personal super-ego, we must recognize the cultural super-ego, as Freud called it.[32]

The elevation of the super-ego to the rank of conscience is the most serious psychologism with which Freud has corrupted man's true conscience. No matter to what a degree we are subject to the authorities of parents and fellow men, we are still free to examine their influence and to decide for ourselves what we consider to be right or wrong. It is true that we have to become aware first of the dependency on others (and we owe Freud the knowledge that such dependency exists), but authoritarian conscience is not true conscience, as Erich Fromm has pointed out.

Personalistic psychologism

Psychologism is not confined to a mechanistic interpretation. Like biologism, it uses general biological concepts in order to account for personal relations. Carl R. Rogers for instance reduces the I-Thou relationship to the level of knowable events. This premise leads not only to a distortion of the essence of personal relationships but also to a distortion of the essence of science.

In his paper 'Persons or Science?' Rogers applies his theory to the relationship between patient and therapist. True to the scientistic foundation, he does not accept that this is a communication between two responsible persons; it is merely an empirical phenomenon which requires for its explanation a scientific hypothesis. In fact, Rogers postulates several scientific hypotheses which have to be 'proved' by objective tests. They are concerned with the regard with which the therapist treats the patient, accepting him as a person, not as an object. This treatment, the hypothesis states, will bring about in the patient a greater feeling of being a person than he had before and 'an experiential and effective type of learning' about himself.[33]

Rogers is, however, not satisfied with the solution which makes the regard and respect of the patient a scientific hypothesis although he was successful in proving 'scientifically' that his patient did benefit from being treated with acceptance. In the second part of his paper he propounds 'a changed view of science'[34] which consists in the assumption that the scientist immerses himself completely in his field and in the relationships which obtain between the phenomena. The confusion of this revised view is worse than the original conception. Rogers takes the 'hunch' which scientists have when they approach the objects of investigation and equates it with the personal subjective faith, which one man has in another. It is of course true that the scientist has faith in his power of observation, in the human intellect, and even in nature's uniformity (which enables him to generalize from a single observation), but none of these 'faiths' have anything to do with the faith which prevails as 'personal subjective faith' in the realm of the I and Thou.[35]

That there is communication between scientists is obvious, and that man has the responsibility to make the correct use of the fruits of scientific research is undoubtedly the case, but we cannot agree that 'science, as well as therapy, as well as all other aspects of living, is rooted in and based upon the immediate, subjective experience of a person'; science *qua* science, is not 'one phase of subjective living',[36] but objective systematized knowledge, based on objective logical principles, objectively valid proofs of evidence, objectively testable theories, and on deductions which have the objective character of universality for the particular field to which they apply. It is therefore misleading when Rogers quotes at the end of his paper the I-Thou relationship, saying that 'science, at its inception, is an "I-Thou" relationship with a person or persons. And only as a subjective person can I enter into either of these relationships'.[37] This distortion of the true position of science and of human communication harms both. Science needs a clear conception of its scope and limitations. The individual person needs a clear view of his scope and limitations in his relations with other persons. The neurosis of our time cannot be overcome if these two issues are blurred.

Evolutionism

Physicalism, biologism, and psychologism annul freedom through extending scientific determinism beyond its legitimate boundaries.

Evolutionism annuls freedom by linking ethics with Darwinian determinism. Evolutionary ethics is a version of humanistic ethics which was criticized earlier on account of the association of ethics with science and with hedonism. Evolutionary ethics is based on a fallacy. C. D. Broad has exposed its logical fault in his *Review of Evolutionary Ethics by Julian S. Huxley,* in which he said: 'unless the notion of value is surreptitiously imported into the definition of "evolution", knowledge of the facts and laws of evolution is simply knowledge of the facts of nature and order of sequence of successive phases in various lines of development'.[38]

The notion of evolution implies continuity of development linking different species in a temporal order. The members of the human species alone are able to distinguish right from wrong. This moral quality is a new phenomenon in the history of evolution: 'it is clearly quite compatible with mere unbrokenness of the temporal sequence to suppose that the development may have exhibited a "new start" more than once. It might be, for instance, that so long as we are dealing with developments within the range of the inorganic, or again within the range of the merely organic, but not conscious, or finally, within the range of the conscious but non-intelligent, we can indicate precisely the connection of each later stage in the development with antecedent changes, accounting for the character of that which appears later completely by the character of what has gone before, but that the first appearance of life, or consciousness, or intelligence, as the case may be, presents us with something definitely *new,* something with a character not fully explicable by reference to anything in the character of what has preceded.'[39]

Darwin himself prepared the ground for the scientism of evolution; for he overlooked the newness of the human mind in the history of evolution, when he referred to 'psychology [as a discipline which] will be securely based on the foundation, already well laid by Mr. Herbert Spencer, that of the necessary acquirement of each mental power and capacity by gradation [and when he added that by such important researches] much light will be thrown on the origin of man and his history'.[40]

Darwin was concerned with the moral issue which his theory raised and tried to make our descent respectable by denigrating the barbarian human ancestor and by elevating the animal forebear. He said: 'For my own part I would as soon be descended from that heroic little monkey, who braced his dreaded enemy in order to save the life of his keeper, or from that old baboon, who descending from the mountains, carried away in triumph his young comrade from a crowd of astonished dogs – as from a savage who delights to torture his enemies, offers up bloody sacrifices, practises infanticide without remorse, treats his wives like slaves, knows no decency, and is haunted by the grossest superstitions.'[41] This argument is confused: our immediate ancestor is the indecent savage and not the heroic monkey or the gallant baboon.

Darwin's tracing of man's moral qualities to the ape is on a par with Freud's account of the evolution of conscience in *Totem and Taboo:* the first stirrings of feelings of guilt and remorse are attributed to the sons of the head of 'the Darwinian original horde' who killed their father, as he had suppressed their desire for power and for sexual satisfaction. They then ate him in order to obtain his strength. This deed is said to have resulted in the awakening of moral feelings as the murderers had in fact harboured ambivalent feelings towards their victim. The logic is wrong: if the sons had not already been endowed with conscience, they would not have felt its stirrings, therefore conscience cannot be derived from the evolutionary movement, apart from the difficulty of placing the origin of conscience accurately within the history of evolution.[42]

Sir Julian Huxley argues in the same vein when he announces: 'We have only recently emerged from the biological to the psychological area of evolution, from the earthly biosphere into the freedom of the noösphere [the sphere of the mind] . . . Our feet still drag in the biological mud, even when we lift our heads into the conscious air. But unlike those remote ancestors of ours, we can truly see something of the promised land beyond. . . We can do so with the aid of our new instrument of vision – our rational, knowledge-based imagination.'[43] The two spheres, one characterized by organic life and the other by a mind which can appreciate the significance of life and is therefore responsible for its own life, that is, which is a moral agent, are different in kind. It is true, of course, that we belong to both spheres; but only a scientism can produce the chimera of one 'science' composed of freedom and of determinism.

Such a union is affirmed in Sir Julian Huxley's writings. He wishes to investigate values, the manifestations of the noösphere, scientifically and asks: 'In what psychological circumstances do values come into being?' The answer is: when man meets his moral obligations. Values must therefore be considered as an expression of man's freedom. Sir Julian Huxley does not accept the ethical interpretation, his reply to this question is confused by his interpretation of values; for he poses a further question: 'Out of what raw materials are they [the values] constructed by man's psycho-metabolic activity?'[44] This question implies a contradiction: the assumption that a deterministic-scientific investigation can explain the dynamics of moral freedom.

Evolutionism makes use of genetics. An authority on this discipline, C. H. Waddington, writes evolutionistically: 'evolution depends. . . on the passing from one generation to the next of something which will determine the character which that following generation will develop'.[45] He goes on to explain the nature of this 'something': the genes, the hereditary units which pass on information and he admits that man 'must take charge of his own evolution'.[46] This is true if Waddington is referring to man's responsibility, but this moral challenge cannot be answered if man's actions, which can determine future evolution, are made a part of the evolutionary process which is said to determine all emerging phenomena.

The confusion of evolutionism is evident in Waddington's contribution to *The Humanist Frame,* as it is in Sir Julian Huxley's. Waddington fails to distinguish between the naturalist-scientific and the ethical points of view in the following statement: 'The basic Humanist position, derived from considering man's place in the biological world, is that in approaching such problems we have to consider them in relation to what we know of the actual *course* of progressive evolution in the sub-human, and in particular of the human world.' In fact, our knowledge of the sub-human part of evolution, our biological knowledge, does not help us; to derive man's responsibility in the shaping of his evolution from his place in the biological world is a fatal error. Evolution is not just 'the very essence of living',[47] as C. H. Waddington holds, and man is not just 'The Human Animal', as his contribution to *The Humanist Frame* is called. The surreptitious introduction of the moral principle within the natural process of evolution is demoralizing, this form of humanism is apt to de-humanize the human being.

Evolutionary humanism, which is based on the fallacy of evolutionary ethics, has recently added to its own confused and confusing evolution by incorporating God in its tenets. The outstanding representative of this school of thought was Pierre Teilhard de Chardin, a Jesuit father, a biologist, and a palaeontologist whose most important book, *The Phenomenon of Man,* has sold many thousands of copies.[48] To the English edition of this work, Sir Julian Huxley has written the Introduction which closely follows the line of thought which has already been criticized.

Teilhard's brand of evolutionary scientism consists in the assertion that the divine element which he called Omega, is the driving force of the whole evolutionary movement, 'the conscious pole' which animates evolution in its lower stages, taking on an impersonal form, using for this purpose 'the veil of biology'. The gist of this thought is not that God is the Creater of the universe or that He inspires biologists whom He has created, but that God takes on the form of biological science and manifests Himself in lower and higher stages. P. W. Medawar is a sharp critic of *The Phenomenon of Man.* He disagrees with the thesis that 'the so-called "psycho-social evolution" of mankind and the genetical evolution of living organisms generally are two episodes of a continuous integral process', and he explains Sir Julian Huxley's handicap which makes it impossible for him to follow Teilhard 'all the way in his gallant attempt to reconcile the supernatural elements in Christianity with the facts and implications of evolution'[49] by demonstrating that the argument of the book is faulty, that it is an attempt to reconcile the irreconcilable, a theological scientism which hinders rather than promotes the gaining of true and much needed faith.[50]

Historicism

Those scientisms which have so far been discussed are derived from the natural sciences. Knowledge of natural phenomena, as we saw, presupposes the assumption of determinism (or causality). This presupposition is, however, not valid for the human personality which is denied its freedom by the unwarranted scientistic extension.

The human being is not only considered as a natural phenomenon, he is also known in terms of a historical process which includes his social setting and the events of his personal history. The examination of social psychiatry demonstrated the failure of the deterministic-causal principle in this branch of psychiatry, although deterministic historical-social factors were admitted. Community psychiatry was described as a form of moral treatment, presupposing human freedom.

By conceiving the human being as a completely determined historical phenomenon, *historicism* adds its corruptive influence to the effects of the other scientisms. In order to clarify the position which determinism plays in the historical personal situation, I shall follow E. P. Papanoutsos' analysis.[51]

In his paper Papanoutsos demonstrates the error of assuming total determinism in the history of a person and thus refutes the notion that we have no freedom and cannot make any decisions in our life. The person who has such a fatalistic outlook is bound to experience life not as his own, but as a process which is beyond his control. Unless he has faith in this controlling power, in a wise and just God, he is liable to find life without sense. Thus the noogenic neurosis of modern man finds a source in the scientism of history.

The historian, Papanoutsos points out, examines events of the past. In contrast to the natural scientist, he does not predict future events, but seeks an explanation by reconstructing them, thus connecting effect with cause and not cause with effect, as is the case in natural science.[52] In a historical, causal examination, the individual person's decision plays a vital part, whereas such freedom has no place in the natural-scientific examination. A person, for instance, who was subjected to the harmful effects of war-time conditions or of economic insecurity in childhood, is not just the product of such conditions. The conduct of his life may well be influenced by the circumstances which prevailed in his childhood, but he has some freedom of choice. The deterministically-orientated psychotherapist is inclined to disregard the true significance of historical causality and to judge the patient's situation according to the faulty conception of historicism, conveying to him the conviction that his previous experiences are the sufficient causes of his present state, thus denying any responsibility and any freedom.

Papanoutsos also stresses the difference between historical time and naturalistic time. The former is non-homogenous and experiential, the latter is homogeneous and neutral so far as subjective experience is concerned.

The experience of time, we found, is also investigated by the phenomenological psychiatrist. He relates such experience to the nosological framework and describes the way in which sufferers from mental illness experience time. The determinism of phenomenological psychology arises from the acceptance of nosological determinism, whereas historical determinism arises from a conception of history as 'a chain of causes and effects with which man is irresistably involved'.[53] Life's meaning depends on the recognition of historical time in its experiential value, and on the allowance made for freedom as an integral part within the framework of reconstructing historical causality.

Objective assessments of the past are necessary for gaining clarity and thus for making sense of a person's life; but objectivity, essential for the conduct of research into natural phenomena, is impossible in the realm of historical phenomena. As W. H. Walsh has pointed out, 'impartial history, so far from being an ideal, is a downright impossibility. . . The work of the historian. . . may be thought to be in some sense an expression of his personality'.[54] Thus in historical assessments, objectivity is relative to a person's subjective point of view. Meaning and purpose are related to the attitude which a particular person adopts towards life. As Walsh admits: 'I must certainly put aside, so far as I can, the moral and metaphysical preconceptions of my own time. But I cannot escape, if I am to make any sense of my material, making some general judgments about human nature, and in these I shall find my own views constantly cropping up. I shall find myself involuntarily shocked by this event and pleased by that, unconsciously seeing this action as reasonable and that as the reverse. And however much I tell myself to eschew my own prejudices and concentrate on understanding what actually happened, I shall not succeed in carrying out the injunction to the latter, since understanding itself is not a passive process, but involves the judging of evidence by principles whose truth is independently assumed.'[55]

W. H. Walsh avoids the danger of historicism by recognizing the impossibility of impartiality and objectivity in the historical judgement. The therapist who is unaware for instance of the correct significance of the sexual or the social trauma in the history of an individual person, and who imagines that he can judge the patient historically-objectively, commits the error of historicism and conveys to the patient the deterministic outlook which denies his freedom and deprives him of the chance of experiencing his life as meaningful.

By expressing his scientistic-fatalistic views in professional and popular writings, this type of scientist corrupts man's striving for freedom and thus intensifies his existential neurosis. Karl Jaspers has pointed out the correct approach, and his words can inspire us to adopt the right attitude towards our history: 'In history we are accessible to ourselves as ourselves. . . in history we encounter ourselves as freedom, as existence, as spirit, as the earnestness of decision, and as independence from the whole world. In history we are addressed by that which does not address us in nature, the mystery of the leaps into liberty, and the manifestations of Being in human consciousness.'[56]

PRESUMPTIONS OF PHENOMENOLOGISM

The cause of freedom is not threatened by the scientists who know and respect the limitations of scientific determinism, as their field is marked off from the field of ethics. Such safeguard does not exist against those philosophers who presume to possess absolute knowledge of Being, of all phenomena, and who incorporate within such a 'science' the freedom of existence which, however, becomes extinct in the framework of an all-embracing phenomenologism. Paradoxically, some of these philosophers are counted amongst the most distinguished and famous existentialists.

Hegel's phenomenologism

Hegel formulated a phenomenology of mind, 'a comprehensive and connected survey of the ways in which experience appears'.[57] Experience is conceived as an unfolding of the objective, universal mind or spirit which understands itself and realizes itself, its highest function being Reason.

The spirit is conscious of itself and consciousness is said to execute on itself the deterministic dialectic process in which the mind becomes an object for itself, leading to a dissimilarity between the ego and the substance which constitutes the object for the ego. This dissimilarity is the factor of negativity.

This negative factor is not only present in the discrepancy between the subject and object, but also finds expression in the inequality of the substance of thought with itself, and as such it becomes the moving principle.

Reason manifests itself as an absolute principle in different forms. The first form is the *in-itself*, the bare abstract form of thought, 'the gazing of the self into the self'. Hegel defines the range of the in-itself as follows: 'It is the mode of self-consciousness which clearly comprehends that in its certainty of self lies the essence of all the component spiritual spheres of the concrete sensible as well as of the supersensible world, or, conversely, that essential being and concrete actuality consist in the knowledge consciousness has of itself.'[58] In other words, the in-itself stands in the Hegelian system for logical systematic thought composed of universal concepts, for 'the ground-plan of the whole of reality, the network of notions which holds together and constitutes the essence of all that is'.[59]

The second form in which absolute Reason appears is the *for-itself*, a manifestation of the spirit in which it comes out of itself, that is, externalizes itself. This self-dispersion again covers 'the whole domain of the Absolute',[60] it is represented by the world of nature, whether inorganic or organic, and is realized in space and time.

The two forms are combined in the *in- and for-itself* which includes pure universality and pure difference, a synthesis 'which avoids these abstract extremes and expresses the concreteness of the Absolute in the highest possible form'.[61]

Hegel affirms rationalism and argues 'that which is reasonable is real, and that which is real is reasonable; thus, reason and reality are identical'. From this premise of identity follows 'that since reason develops, the world must develop, and since the development of thought or reason is a dialectic one, the world must also develop in dialectic triads' [of thesis, antithesis and synthesis].[62]

An impartial critic cannot accept the principle of identity. As K. R. Popper says, Hegel's philosophy is dogmatic and a 'panlogism'; it presumes to equate reality with logical thought; in other words, it makes thought processes into entities and assumes that these entities exist in an objective manner. His error is hypostatization, making something real which exists only in the mind.

Hegel's dogmatic approach has been taken over by Sartre in a modified way, and forms an integral part of his existential philosophy. In view of Sartre's profound influence on people, his phenomenologism will now be examined.

Sartre's phenomenologisms

As Sartre's views on man's situation have changed markedly in the course of his life, it is necessary to discuss his earlier formulations separately from his later exposition.

Sartre's first version of phenomenologism

Sartre took over Hegel's hypostatized concepts *in-itself, for-itself* and *negativity* and related them to each other as a deterministic dialectic process. His definitions of these concepts in *Being and Nothingness* are as follows: the for-itself is the conscious subject which can separate itself from being and is thus a manifestation of freedom. The in-itself is the non-conscious being, something inhuman. The principle of negativity is invested in the for-itself as an internal negation of consciousness. As in the case of Hegel's phenomenologism, negativity is the moving principle: 'the for-itself arises as the nihilation of the in-itself'. As freedom is the ability to project, to find a goal, to choose being, in cases where there had been lack of being, 'the for-itself is the being which is to itself its own lack of being [and] the being which the for-itself lacks is the in-itself'.[63]

What is the meaning and significance of this interpretation of the human situation? The Sartrian man finds himself in a desperate dilemma and in an insoluble conflict which has all the elements for an effective drama on the stage or for a plot in a novel; the validity of the dilemma must, however, be rejected because of its phenomenologistic character. The predicament of the Sartrian man does not arise from a genuine conflict, but from a constellation of the pieces of Hegel's dialectic which have been given a new connotation. Man's reality has been constructed by the metaphysician Sartre, and the playwright and novelist Sartre contrives his plots according to the metaphysical, phenomenologistic plan. The existentialist Sartre upholds the idea of freedom and makes man responsible for his deeds, but how can this poor man meet his responsibilities and cope with his life? In order to answer this question, let us compare the Sartrian with the Hegelian man.

Whereas Hegel's phenomenologism inspires man by presenting his history as an unfolding of his free spirit, Sartre's phenomenologism crushes his hope by depriving freedom of its essence; for freedom is not part of human existence, it precedes it and makes existence possible. Man is thus free, but he lacks the freedom not to be free, he is therefore condemned to be free. The situation of the free for-itself is so desperate because the in-itself, which for Hegel was one of the manifestations of the free spirit, has been turned into a thing without freedom. Unfortunately, the in-itself takes precedence over the for-itself ontologically and essentially. The in-itself wins over the for-itself: 'Thus the end and the goal of the nihilation which I am is the in-itself.'[64] Thus human existence becomes absurd.

The Sartrian man not only lives in a world of despair, he is also deprived of the chance to be a sincere person. The Sartrian dialectic sabotages the aim of sincerity by identifying it with the aim of insincerity; bad faith is inevitable: 'In order for me to have an intention of sincerity, I must at the outset simultaneously be and not be what I am. . . Bad faith requires that I should not be what I am. . . it attempts also to constitute myself as being what I am not. . . If it were not on principle impossible for me to coincide with my not-being-courageous as well as with my being-courageous – then any project of bad faith would be prohibited me.'[65]

Sartre's conclusion follows from deriving human existence from his concepts of being-in-itself and being-for-itself, but, as Gabriel Marcel has pointed out in answer to this piece of Sartrian sophistry, sincerity in fact does not presuppose the determinism of being, but the freedom of becoming, namely of becoming a different person.[66]

The unhappy Sartrian man suffers a further blow as the result of the adoption of the dogmatic ontological-phenomenologistic framework: he is isolated from his fellow human beings. The argument runs as follows: a man's freedom is his subjectivity, which is also his consciousness. This freedom is lost if he becomes the object of somebody else's consciousness: 'If somebody looks at me, I am conscious of being an object. . . The other does not constitute me an object for myself but for him. . . [therefore] my freedom is alienated in the presence of the Other's pure subjectivity which founds my objectivity.'[67] Hence mutual hate and suspicion amongst men, in fact paranoia, are inevitable: 'The Other flees me when I seek him and possesses me when I flee him. . . While I attempt to free myself from the hold of the Other, the Other is trying to free himself from mine; while I seek to enslave the Other, the Other seeks to enslave me.'[68] The follower of personalistic existential ethics who strives for I-Thou relations must protest against the paranoid conception of human existence that 'Hell is. . . other people'.[69]

Sartre's phenomenologistic view of human relations has influenced R. D. Laing. Laing is less pessimistic than Sartre, as he admits that 'one may find oneself enlivened and the sense of one's own being enhanced by the other'. Nobody can deny that 'one may experience the other as deadening and impoverishing', even that one may be 'threatened with the possibility of becoming no more than a thing in the world of the other, without any life for oneself, without any being for oneself', but this possibility does not arise, as Laing (following Sartre) maintains, from becoming an object of awareness in somebody else's consciousness. The risk of dehumanization does not 'consist in this: if one experiences the other as a free agent, one is open to the possibility of experiencing oneself as an *object* of his experience and thereby of feeling one's own subjectivity drained away'.[70] On the contrary, the experience of free people of each other leads to the mutual confirmation of their subjectivity and of their freedom.

Sartre's second version of phenomenologism

The account of man's freedom, of his striving for sincerity and for relations with other men, which Sartre derived from Hegel's phenomenologism, was followed by the adoption of another phenomenologism which was based on the Marxian doctrine.

The emphasis is now on social determinism. An example is Sartre's *Saint Genet,* summarized and commented on by R. D. Laing and D. G. Cooper in *Reason and Violence.* The individual is alleged to lose his freedom; 'the social actions of a person are conditioned by the general interests of his class',[71] because of the dialectic process between him and social-historical reality. Genet serves as an example of this kind of determinism.

Genet was caught stealing as a child and was identified by society as a thief. This act by the 'honest' people is said to follow the law according to which they project their wickedness on a scapegoat. Genet's freedom lies in his decision 'to be what the others had made him to be'.[72] (Sartre goes beyond the Marxian dialectic by assuming a further dialectic between freedom and fate.)

R. D. Laing's interpretation of the schizophrenic's case corresponds closely to Sartre's interpretation of Genet's case. Laing says: 'There is no such "condition" as "schizophrenia", but the label is a social fact and the social fact a *political event.* This political event, occurring in the civic order of society, imposes definitions and consequences on the labelled person. It is a social prescription that rationalizes a set of social actions whereby the labelled person is annexed by others, who are legally sanctioned, medically empowered, and morally obliged, to become responsible for the person labelled. The person labelled is inaugurated not only into a role, but into a career of patient, by the concerted action of a coalition (a "conspiracy") of family G.P., mental health officer, psychiatrists, nurses, psychiatric social workers, and often fellow patients.'[73]

There is a parallelism between the case of Genet and the case of the schizophrenic: both are weak personalities (Genet's weakness was due to the fact that society brought its influence to bear on him when he was a child). Society is strong in comparison with the individual, but is itself weak, suffering from the malaise of a general uncertainty of values. This weakness finds a reflection in the minds of the schizophrenic and the criminal. The treatment of these individuals labelled as sick or delinquents follows, of course, different lines. In the case of the criminal, society has to protect itself. In the case of the schizophrenic, certain protective measures are also often necessary. Most of Laing's criticisms are directed against these measures.

Laing is unfair in implying that all hospital staff act inhumanly against the patient at the behest of society, just as only certain individual members of society lack the appreciation of another person's freedom and thus contribute to his mental breakdown. Such human failings are not the failings of society as a whole.

While people with weak mental constitutions and children admittedly succumb easily to the influence of society, healthy adult people can resist social pressure. The Marxian-Sartrian phenomenologism denies such freedom of the individual. In his *Critique of Dialectical Reason* (also distilled by R. D. Laing and D. G. Cooper in *Reason and Violence*) Sartre pictures man as 'totalized by the mode of production'.[74] He gives the following example of a socio-economic nexus: 'The life-course of a worker at Dop Shampoos, even down to the fantasies of the machinist, is predetermined in general. The factory girl, in her sexual relations, pregnancies, abortions, *realizes* by herself what she is *already*. She passes against herself the sentence already passed by the whole nexus of socio-economic conditions into which she has been born.'[75]

The denial of freedom which follows from Marxian phenomenologism must be rejected. The factory worker must be granted the freedom to resist the pressure from society. Dialectical materialism is no more valid than dialectical idealism.

Husserl's phenomenologism

The dogmatic phenomenologistic interpretations of consciousness by Hegel, Marx, and his followers are one source of confusion, the other source lies in Husserl's interpretation of consciousness. As Husserl has had a strong influence on a number of existential psychiatrists and on the existential philosophy of Martin Heidegger, his phenomenologism merits special attention.

Husserl's phenomenological approach went through different stages which Stephen Strasser has surveyed in a paper entitled 'Phenomenologies and Psychologies'.[76]

Husserl's descriptive psychological phenomenology

Husserl's starting point was a descriptive psychological phenomenology which coincides with the approach of phenomenological psychiatry, based, as we said, on the data of consciousness, that is, on the (inner) subjective world of experience. These data have reality for the particular person and must be respected by the psychiatrist. (The question of their reality apart from the individual's consciousness does not arise.)

Karl Jaspers was the first psychiatrist who applied Husserl's descriptive phenomenological method to the understanding of his patients. Other psychiatrists such as von Gebsattel, Minkowski, and Binswanger have enriched our knowledge of the different worlds in which mental patients live (see the reference to these investigations in the section on phenomenological psychiatry.[77]) These empirical observations do not cancel out the individual's freedom, but point to the limitations which are due to his illness. He can still realize some of his potentialities even in a world of depression, of schizophrenia, of obsessional neurosis or of any other mental disorder.

Husserl's transcendental phenomenologism

Husserl left the realm of descriptive psychological phenomenology and abandoned the 'natural' empirical standpoint. Through intuitive perception, he claimed to reach the 'sphere of essences', 'the eidetically observable' which were mentioned in the discussion of freedom in relation to the inner world. This road, he maintained, led to transcendence, understood as 'an immanent, constituting character of being, within the ego itself', that is, within consciousness;[78] his goal was the *a priori* of an absolute eidetic science.

Husserl was convinced that he had reached his goal, but we cannot follow him in this transcendental endeavour, as it leads to such arbitrary ontologies as Sartre's formulations in *Being and Nothingness.*

Hallucinations as eidetic phenomena

An example of an unacceptable transcendental phenomenologism is the paper by Dick Howard, entitled 'Hallucination: A Phenomenological Analysis'.[79] This writer accepts Aldous Huxley's claim to have discovered new frontiers of the mind through having taken mescalin, as this drug produces 'true' hallucinations, characterized by a 'perceptual' character, 'appearing in objective space and time usually in a vivid and clearly delineated manner', whereas 'pseudo-hallucinations' are lacking 'the character of objectivity, possessing 'a certain character of subjectivity, especially in that they appear in inner subjective space'.[80] Apart from mescalin, Howard mentions LSD and alcohol as giving rise to true hallucinations, alcohol when it causes delirium tremens.

The connection between true hallucinations and Husserl's transcendental phenomenology is explained in the following way: Husserl taught that consciousness is intentional, by which he meant that it always aimed at something (we are always conscious of something). The hallucination is one of the targets of the intention, 'the product of an objectivating intentionality'. Thus pathological states of the mind which arise from the taking of drugs become experiences of 'primordial givenness', illuminated by 'the ray of consciousness', revealing a new level of the mind: 'When the hallucinatory quality appears, there is new depth added.'

The road which Dick Howard praises leads to the mystique of Timothy Leary which has attracted thousands of people, especially the young. They have escaped into the transcendental realm. Their 'expanding' minds have lost touch with the reality side of consciousness and they have become unfit for ordinary life.

Whereas Dick Howard excludes the psychotic experience from the field of 'primal' experiences, R. D. Laing looks to the schizophrenic experience as the true reality with which the so-called normal person has lost contact.[81]

We must reject the notion that the transcendental can be reached through intoxication and must deny the validity of Dick Howard's argument and of the premise, which is implied in Husserl's transcendental phenomenologism. We must relate experience to conscience and measure the significance of the emotional phenomenon by its contribution to the achievement of a more mature form of authentic existence.

Heidegger's phenomenologism

Husserl claimed that 'a systematically developed transcendental phenomenology would be the true and genuine universal Ontology'.[82] He held that such ontology was inherent in consciousness. Heidegger deviated from Husserl by establishing an alleged ontology independent of consciousness. He delineated a field of Being as such, of man's Being. His phenomenologism has been acclaimed as true by psychiatrists such as M. Boss, and has been made the foundation for their approach to the patient; and we met this type of phenomenologism in J. F. T. Bugental's definition of authenticity as 'an ultimate state of at-oneness with the cosmos'.[83]

Heidegger's phenomenology is acceptable only as a contribution to descriptive psychological phenomenology. He draws attention to important aspects of the human situation. It is true that man has to come to terms with his death and with the experience of nothingness, and that the crowd tends to prevent him from facing such tasks and from achieving authenticity. Heidegger reminds us that we have been thrown into the world where we are liable to feel lost, and that the feeling of dread which we experience in our lonely struggle can open our eyes to our possibilities. Heidegger's ontological claims must, however, be rejected as phenomenologistic. The difference between the two interpretations of his philosophy is of decisive importance for the sufferer from the existential neurosis as the following examples show.

Man has to accept the experience of nothing as a challenge which has to be faced. Human existence is, however, not nothingness, as Heidegger maintains. Although he affirms man's freedom to be his own self and stresses the importance of his freedom to choose, he denigrates the freedom to choose through introducing the principle of nullity: choosing implies the need to reject the alternative which has not been chosen, and such a rejection is in fact a moral victory for the person; to Heidegger, man is guilty, as he can choose only one possibility.

Heidegger and Sartre, two outstanding existential philosophers, have shaken modern man by their presentations of his predicament. These presentations are false and misleading on account of their phenomenologistic basis. They tend to prevent the sufferers from the existential neurosis from gaining the freedom of their existence.

FAITH OF IRRATIONALISM

Phenomenologisms and scientisms are abuses of the ratio which has its legitimate use in science and in logical thought. We must ask whether the ethical philosophy advocated in this book is rational and, if the reply is negative, whether its irrational character makes it into an unconvincing or mystical or romantic interpretation of life. Its existential basis provides the clue to this problem.

As D. E. Roberts has pointed out, existentialism 'is a protest against all forms of rationalism which find it easy to assume that reality can be grasped primarily or exclusively by intellectual means. It is an emphatic denial of the assumption that construction of a logical system is the most adequate way to reach the truth'.[84]

What is the truth proclaimed by personalistic existential ethics? We saw that it is the truth of personal conscience which demands of everyone the utmost use of his freedom. Conscience is not irrational; in Kantian terminology, it is, on the contrary, the expression of practical reason (whereas science represents an expression of theoretical reason).

While the categorical imperative which tells each man to do his duty (towards himself and others) is a rational principle which can be grasped by intellectual means, the individuality of man and of his world of experience cannot be so grasped.

Martin Buber has clarified the nature and the realm of the irrational. In his essay 'With a Monist', he contrasted the monistic rationalistic conception with the view which allows for irrationality. The former standpoint reduces all phenomena to the level of a universal principle, it comprehends the world. The latter holds that 'all comprehensibility of the world is only a footstool of its incomprehensibility'.[85]

Incomprehensibility in Buber's sense is, however, not just negative. On the contrary, the person who knows the world outside or within himself without the use of his ratio gathers far richer knowledge than he can obtain with the aid of the rational principle: 'What the most learned and ingenious combination of concepts denies, the humble and faithful beholding, grasping, knowing of any situation bestows. The world is not comprehensible, but it is embraceable: through the embracing of one of its beings.' As Buber has said 'each thing and being has a twofold nature: the passive, absorbable, usable, dissectible, comparable, combinable, rationalizable, and the other, the active, non-absorbable, unusable, undissectible, incomparable, noncombinable, nonrationalizable.'[86]

Modern man whose mind has been steeped in rationalism must become aware of the significance of irrationalism which opens the way to that world which is closed to the rational approach. His own personality and his fellow human beings, the qualities of the inner and outer worlds, and the significance of the voice of conscience can be grasped only by means of the irrational standpoint.

The acceptance of the irrational principle does not imply a turning away from reality in mystical denial and negation. On the contrary, by adopting the non-rational attitude, man confronts the world and the people in it, and the world discloses its meaning to him.

The gaining of faith depends on the ability to face the world irrationally, to hold oneself open 'to the unconditional mystery which we encounter in every sphere of our life and which cannot be comprised in any formula... Real faith means the ability to endure life in the face of this mystery. The forms in which the mystery approaches us are nothing but our personal experiences.'[87]

Irrationality, understood in Buber's sense, is thus not opposed to reason. By means of the irrational approach, man can gain clarity (although not the clarity of conceptual science), faith in himself and in the world, and freedom from the existential neurosis.

Treatment

5

The Existential Position

We arrived at the diagnosis of the neurotic malaise which we recognized as a crisis in valuation, a moral phenomenon. As an ethical (and not a scientific) approach was needed to deal with the critical situation, we investigated first traditional moral philosophies, which we found unsuitable for our purpose as they are merely theoretical systems without any concern for the results which their acceptance has for the holder of a particular moral philosophy. Humanistic ethics, put forward as a substitute for religious faith, and by Erich Fromm as a basis for psychotherapy, was rejected because of its deterministic-scientific foundation and its hedonistic fallacy. We then examined Viktor E. Frankl's psychiatrically-orientated ontological value ethic which was unacceptable because of its inconsistencies. Finally, an answer was proposed which affirms the freedom of existence and relates a person's authenticity to his transcendence. Freedom, we saw, can be realized in a man's 'inner' world of experience and in his 'outer' world, when he communicates with his fellow men and undertakes creative activities. The freedom of decision was interpreted as a test for his faith in which, alas, the neurotic is lacking. For him, there are no guiding principles on which decisions could be based. Therefore he is frightened to commit himself, but he cannot escape from his responsibilities without feeling guilty. His conscience demands of him the fulfilment of his obligations towards himself and others.

Some limitations of freedom were admitted as inevitable, but human bondage was found to be aggravated as the result of unwarranted presumptions which are made by proclaimers of scientisms and phenomenologisms and which confuse and corrupt people. At the end of the last chapter, the irrational character of the underlying philosophy was clarified as being the attitude which enables man to become aware of the meaning of life.

EXISTENTIAL NEUROSIS

Personalistic existential ethics was outlined as a blueprint for existential psychotherapy and we must now apply its principles to the treatment of actually sick people, to sufferers from the noogenic neurosis. An account of the struggle for freedom of individual patients will, it is hoped, not only elucidate the ethical theory of this book, but will also provide an inspiration to those who search for a personal, practical solution of their crisis in valuation. In the following discussion, the term 'existential' will designate the author's specific meaning which distinguishes it from the way it is used by other existential writers.

6

Approach to the Patient

Existential psychotherapy relies on the moral resources of the patient. It aims at mobilizing these forces by providing them with a target. It presupposes that, dissatisfied with his state of inauthenticity, he is prepared to meet the challenges of his existence in order to increase his freedom. The existential therapist therefore has to choose methods of treatment which put the patient face to face with his task.

METHODS OF EXISTENTIAL CONFRONTATION

Man gains freedom from bondage by facing his restrictions and himself. A therapist can assist a patient in his striving for freedom by confronting him with his situation and with the possibilities of self-liberation.

Numerous methods are available for existential confrontation. We shall now survey some of the techniques which existential therapists can employ, but these must not be considered apart from the aim of the treatment, which is the gaining of freedom.

The interview

People obtain clarity by looking at their situation with somebody else, by interviews. They feel encouraged to verbalize their thoughts when they meet someone whom they can trust and who is interested in their affairs. He may be a relative or a friend, and existential therapy has been carried out since time immemorial by those who care for their fellow human beings in distress. While the trained therapist has no monopoly of existential therapy, he has qualifications which distinguish him from the non-professional person. These qualifications will be discussed later.

The patient attains a view of his life by telling the therapist his story, going back to his earliest childhood, relating his emotional development, and gaining insight into the factors and circumstances which prevented him from achieving his freedom.

In listening to the patient, the therapist forms an opinion of the patient's dissatisfaction with himself, his motivation to change, and his strength to achieve a more authentic existence. The initial interview enables him to plan the treatment and further meetings serve to develop the plan.

The interviews need not be restricted to a meeting of therapist and one person. Frequently, the emotional situation can be clarified only if all those who participate in it, that is, several members of a family, meet the therapist (the fruitfulness of such sessions depends on the motivation of all concerned, often only the patient who has broken down shows the necessary initiative).

Individual psychotherapy provides the patient with a chance of forming a relationship with the therapist which involves, however, the risk of dependency, that is, of lack of freedom. This danger can be lessened if patients meet the therapist in a group.

Existential group therapy is not concerned with group dynamics, with the clarification of the objective, interpersonal processes. Such studies are undertaken by therapists who accept the framework of scientific, objective determinism. As the existential therapist is guided by the idea of freedom, his aim is to help the members of the group to realize their potentialities through personal communication and to face their personal limitations.

The therapeutic group consists of a small number of people who meet their therapist regularly. A larger circle gives people the advantage of social life which many lack because of their neurotic restrictions. The therapeutic social club is particularly helpful; it provides opportunities for discussion, for informal personal meetings, and all sorts of activities such as dancing, playing table tennis, and so on; in such a club people feel accepted, which helps them to become confident. Such experience is essential for the gaining of personal freedom.[1]

Dream interpretation

By meeting the therapist and other patients, people can gain insight into their situation. They can see their tasks even more clearly with the aid of messages received from the unconscious. Existential therapists make use of the technique of free association which was developed by Freud. It is in their interpretation that they differ from him.

Dream interpretation plays an important part in the Freudian and in the existential approach, as dreams are communications from the unconscious. The existential therapist agrees with Freud that some dreams contain 'unmistakably the realisation of a desire',[2] but would differ by adding that such a desire implies a challenge and by confronting the dreamer with the task of facing the desire. Some of Freud's examples can serve to illustrate the difference between the two approaches; for instance, the dream of a young woman who wished to meet again a man whom she had last met at the funeral of her sister's eldest child. She thus dreamt of the second child's death without feeling pain, but also without feeling pleasure (as she is struggling against her desire).[3] The existentialist would (like the Freudian) uncover the woman's longing, but would encourage her to come to terms with it and with its implications.

According to Freud, some dreams do not express any wish-fulfilment, but refer to either real or imagined terrifying sexual experience in childhood. In such dreams, intercourse is symbolized by a violent act, for instance a murder (to the child who has witnessed the parents' intercourse, violence is the keynote of the experience).[4]

The existential therapist agrees that such an experience is a shock to the patient and that he must re-live it in order to overcome its effects. A violent dream may be associated in his mind with a violent sexual scene. The existentialist encourages such a person to face the various forms of violence which he has experienced. He does not, however, agree with Freud that violence is a primary instinctual urge (whether associated with the sexual urge or not), but sees in it a challenge to a person's freedom and assists him to deal with the challenge.

A comparison with the Jungian conception of dreams can clarify the existential standpoint further. Gerhard Adler, a follower of Jung, reported the following dream of an over-ambitious business man: 'It is harvest time; I am sitting on a large wagon, laden with hay, which I am driving back to the barn, but the load of hay is so high that the lintel of the door. . . knocks me on the head, so that I fall off my seat and I wake up terrified.' Adler saw in this dream a warning from this man's unconscious: he should compensate for his overdeveloped extraversion by developing his 'inner need'.[5]

The barn is taken to be a manifestation of the mother-archetype and the conclusion is reached that the patient is not only fixated to and frightened by his personal mother (for whom the barn, a womb-like structure, is also a symbol), but is also faced with 'the deeper problem of the relationship to the mother-archetype. . . this. . . the first form of the anima-experience'.[6]

The existential therapist does not accept the Jungian framework. To him, a dream is a message from a personal unconscious; it is thus subjective. The objective element in the existential approach lies in the acknowledgement of the moral principle which, however, is not expected to work according to any set rules. The therapist deciphers a particular dream message by asking the patient to tell him what comes to his mind in relation to the various features of the dream.

The existentialist agrees with the Jungian that the dream quoted by Gerhard Adler indicates a danger to the dreamer, a loss of balance. Through the process of association, the particular nature of the danger would have to be discovered and faced. In coping with it, man is neither seen as threatened by dangerous archetypes (as Jungian patients are said to be) nor is he considered as gaining help from 'the self-regulating', 'objective psyche'.[7]

'Reverie' technique

If a patient cannot remember his dreams, the therapist can confront him with his tasks through the induction of a dream-like 'reverie'. In this condition, a person can communicate with his therapist on a deeper level than when he is in the ordinary wakeful state.

The patient must be prepared for the treatment and must be re-assured by the therapist with regard to the alteration of consciousness. Then the therapist suggests relaxation of the whole body and can, in suitable subjects, hypnotize the patient, but relaxation with closure of eyes is sufficient. He is now ready for the reverie: he is told that he is in a theatre facing the stage. After he has confirmed that he can see the stage, he is asked to describe the performance.

The drama which follows is the drama of the patient's life. Often scenes from the actual past, especially his childhood, are enacted. The patient sees himself in critical situations and re-lives the tension and anxiety which he could not face at the time and which has crippled him.

Some patients dramatize their present conflicts by means of phantastic figures: monsters, devils, knights in shining armour, and so on. As in dream interpretation, the significance of these symbols for the particular person's existence is discovered through the process of association, but the confrontation in the reverie can be made more effective than the discussion of a dream; for the patient faces his problem while in the reverie and can play out the solution with the therapist acting as a producer or as a member of the cast. The session is terminated with general assurance.

After a person has learnt the reverie technique he can carry out this form of treatment by himself and can discuss his reveries with his therapist during his next consultation.[8]

Drawings and paintings

Apart from dreams and reveries, free drawings and paintings are expressions of the unconscious. By confronting patients with these products of their imagination (which are not interpreted as works of art), the therapist can provide and gain further insight into their worlds of experience.

Painting (or drawing) can form part of the programme of the therapeutic social club. On the evening set aside for this activity, patients are encouraged to draw whatever comes to their minds. After about thirty minutes the drawings are put up for all members of the club to see, and the therapist then asks those present to give their interpretations for each picture. He writes their comments on the margin of the drawing, and these can be used, together with the picture itself, as material for the following individual session. Some patients draw scenes from their past or present life, others express their emotional situation abstractly in a few lines with a few colours.

Mental health films

A patient's drawing, his reverie, and his dream are products of his own phantasy, but he can be stirred also by the products of other people's imagination, for instance, by so-called mental health films, which are particularly suitable for an audience such as the members of a therapeutic social club.

Some films depict the problems of childhood. They can help people to re-live their own early life and to see their present difficulties in the light of these memories. A good example which brings to mind the pains of growing-up is 'Farewell to Childhood'. The central character is a girl aged fifteen. Her parents do not grasp the emotional problems of their adolescent daughter, her untidiness, and emotional instability. The therapist is seen to help the girl to gain understanding from her parents and freedom to grow up. 'Preface to Life' highlights the danger of a possessive mother, who makes her son feel guilty when he wants to be independent, and the significance of a father's ambition for his boy.

'Roots of Happiness' brings home the unhappy situation in a Puerto Rican family living in overcrowded conditions, the father bullying his wife and children and the mother feeling resentful. This situation is contrasted with one of a happy family in which parents and children have enough room to develop and in which everybody is treated with consideration. In this film many people discover the roots of their own unhappiness. 'Angry Boy' expresses the violence of a generally disturbed child who has become a thief. He works through his problems with the aid of a psychiatrist while his mother is seen gaining insight into her own attitudes. The boy's anger can release the same feelings in the audience, which can be helped to face the sources and manifestations of their own aggressiveness.

The subject of hostility is treated from another angle in 'The Feelings of Hostility'. In this drama there is no outburst of violence, but a coldness in a girl who has lacked a warm relationship with her mother. The girl finds a professional outlet for her ability, but she cannot love people and is therefore a lonely person. This film provides a great deal of material for discussion, as many withdrawn patients identify themselves with the main character. Hostility arises when a person feels rejected. This situation is well brought out in the film 'The Feeling of Rejection': a young woman who has been exploited by everybody learns to stand up to the unreasonable demands from her family and her fellow workers and to overcome her resentment.

Rejection can lead to depression, as the rejected person loses the strength to cope with life. Another film, 'Feelings of Depression', demonstrates how early emotional deprivation can bring about depression. The man, the main character, becomes unable to carry out his work, but he finds his way back into life with the aid of psychotherapy. Many immature patients are kept in a state which the film 'Over Dependency' depicts. It is the story of a young man who leans on his mother, sister, and wife. The doctor makes him realize that he has not faced life and helps him to find a more mature attitude. An elderly widow finds it hard not to lean on her married children; this problem is illustrated in 'Steps of Age'. Both the widow and her married daughter gain insight into the problems of their lives and into their mutual relationship.

These examples illustrate the part which the showing of mental health films can play in existential therapy. The discussion which follows the film enables patients to express their feelings and to recognize their own situation through an exchange of views.

Mental health films have also been helpful in the field of mental hygiene. Milton Miles Berger has described this form of health education. He found that the audiences (up to two hundred people) are stimulated by the films 'to discuss their own personal values, attitudes and problems'.[9] People who are afraid to consult a psychiatrist often attend these meetings which have been arranged for 'normal' people. The questions asked by the sick person frequently prove to be particularly helpful in the discussion.

Use of drugs

The encounters with the personalities of therapist and fellow patients, with their own dreams and reveries, and with the characters of mental health films are strong stimulants of the existential forces in the inauthentic person, but they may not be powerful enough. A drug may be required to initiate an experience which enables the self to gain insight into its situation and which stimulates it to strive for its freedom.

The therapist must be aware of the dangers of using drugs as aids to his treatment. Drug addiction, we have seen, is one of the manifestations of neurosis. The addict seeks drug experience in order to avoid facing himself and his life situation. The existential therapist is justified in using drugs only if he has satisfied himself that his patient will use the drug experience as a means of realizing his freedom and not of avoiding it.

The following types of drugs can be employed as aids to existential psychotherapy.

Amylobarbitone (Sodium Amytal)

Amylobarbitone, given intravenously in doses of 125 mg or 250 mg, relaxes a patient and can free his mind for the tasks of his existence. It can be combined with a cerebral stimulant.

Methylamphetamine (Methedrine)

Methylamphetamine is a powerful stimulant of the nervous system and is particularly liable to lead to addiction. The therapist who gives methylamphetamine at intervals of two or three weeks to a patient intravenously can, however, judge whether the patient develops a craving for this substance and can then stop further administration in time.

Methylphenidate Hydrochloride (Ritalin)

Methylphenidate hydrochloride is another cerebral stimulant. Its effect is similar to that of methylamphetamine but wears off more rapidly, so that the patient can leave the consulting room within one hour. As with other stimulants, there is the danger of addiction.

Lysergic Acid Diethylamide (LSD) 25

LSD 25 does not cause addiction. It can, however, become the means of escaping into a world of unreality, as was pointed out when the abuses of Husserl's transcendental phenomenalism were discussed. In addition, LSD 25 has produced outbursts of violence, acting out of suicidal and homicidal impulses, and has precipitated attacks of depression and psychotic breakdowns. Because of such dangers, the therapist must satisfy himself that the patient is strong enough to cope with the drug experience.

A further hazard was reported in 1967 when M. M. Cohen and his co-workers discovered chromosome damage in LSD users.[10] Other workers demonstrated the same effects from other drugs including aspirin and caffeine. D. A. Hungerford in association with five scientists evaluated this hazard. They showed that chromosome abnormalities were transitory and no longer evident after one month. They concluded that LSD 25 is as safe as many other commonly used drugs.[11]

The existential therapist does not administer LSD for the sake of producing hallucinatory experiences. He does not accept experience *per se* as a worthwhile aim and does not send his patients on 'trips' into a psychedelic world for kicks. (In the section on Husserl's transcendental phenomenologism the interpretation of hallucinatory experiences as desirable eidetic phenomena in the Husserlian sense was rejected.)

Although LSD has pharmacological properties, the experience of LSD intoxication lies outside the realm of objective science. It is a methodological mistake to subject such experience to objective criteria as H. J. Eysenck did in his review of *The Varieties of Psychedelic Experience* by R. E. L. Masters and J. Houston. Eysenck, writing in *Medical News,* criticized the book because the claims from users of LSD had 'no empirical foundation whatever'. In so far as such claims relate to skills which can be tested, Eysenck may be right in insisting on objective checks, but to the extent to which they relate to coping better with life – and this is the whole point of Masters and Houston's book – 'experimental' evidence cannot be expected. Eysenck admitted in his review that the moral claim which is made by writers of the book 'is hardly subject to empirical demonstration'. How true!

The moral issue cannot be settled by scientific research, it is the central issue for modern man who has lost faith. The experience which LSD provides can enable individual patients to face their moral problems, to grasp the potentialities of their lives, and to accept responsibilities.

LSD should be used only after the therapist has established firm communication with the patient and has assured himself that the patient has the motivation to face his responsibilities. While the patient is under the influence of LSD, the therapist must be with him, interpreting the various experiences in terms of existential ethics. The therapist's presence is also essential to sustain the patient while he faces the often shattering revival of childhood traumata, the hallucinatory visions and voices, and while he goes through agony and hope and transcendental experiences of different kinds. The following account of an LSD session illustrates the depth of this treatment.

> I felt as if I was being split open and turned inside out, as if the edges of the cut were curling outwards, trying to make what was inside me come out. It was terrifying. Although I was very

frightened, never having experienced anything like this before, I sensed somehow that it was absolutely necessary for me to go through the experience, to give myself up to my fear.

This patient went through similar anxiety four times during one LSD session. She reported that after the fourth time, the terror got less. The changes which she felt in the course of this session are significant: 'each time I went into the experience, I was able to go further into it, giving myself up to it a little more, although my fear and the pain were still terrible'. The result of this treatment was that she felt more alive. She realized that she had been in 'a terrible vice' all her life and longed to get out of it. No other method could have given her the opportunity and courage to achieve her aim.

LSD can be combined with methylamphetamine and with methylphenidate hydrochloride. Chlorpromazine counteracts LSD and can be given to terminate its action.

The existential therapist can combine the different methods. A patient who has received a drug will often become a more active member of a therapeutic social club or a group or will benefit more from individual sessions.

THE THERAPEUTIC ENCOUNTER

Existential psychotherapy depends on certain techniques which enable the patients to come to grips with their inauthenticity, with their lack of freedom; but the techniques are not the essential element. The personal encounter between the patient, his therapist, and other patients is the vital factor.

Buber's account of the I-Thou relationship which was quoted in the exposition of the personalistic existential ethic provides us with the framework for the understanding of the therapeutic encounter. Especially illuminating is his description of the person who does not relate to the world: he becomes incapsulated and develops on himself, 'on the unnatural, impossible object of the I. . . where there is no place at all. . . to develop'.[13] To reverse this unhappy situation is the aim of the therapeutic encounter.

Buber defined the conditions which must be fulfilled for the liberation of the patient as follows: 'The real matter, the regeneration of an atrophied personal centre. . . can only be done by one who grasps the buried latent unity of the suffering soul with the great glance of the doctor: and this can only be attained in the person-to-person attitude of a partner.'[14]

Complete mutuality which characterizes the relationship of equal partners does not apply in the therapeutic encounter. As Buber has pointed out, the therapist has to feel with the patient apart from having his own feelings. 'In order that he may coherently further the liberation and actualisation of that unity in a new accord of the person with the world, the psychotherapist, like the educator, must stand again and again not merely at his own pole in the bipolar relationship, but also with the strength of present realisation at the other pole, and experience the effect of his own action.'[15]

As C. A. Seguin has pointed out, the relationship between the therapist and the patient represents a special form of love, different from the love between friends, relatives, and lovers. Psychotherapeutic love, which is the basis of existential therapy, has nothing to do with authority and possessiveness, with identification, with dogma, with imposition of values, of rules, or of knowledge, and must be devoid of sexual feelings.[16] It must be indestructible.[17] Therapeutic love carries the therapist forward in his efforts to reach the patient, it is the force which causes in the sufferer a reorientation, a change of polarity.

Buber explained in his dialogue with Carl R. Rodgers what he meant by polarity. The two poles represent acceptance and refusal, yes and no.[18] The positive pole is said to stand for direction and order, the negative pole for lack of direction and for chaos.

The emotionally disturbed person is in a chaotic state, the therapist relies on the innate wish for a more orderly state and on the capacity to achieve this end. The sick person wants and requires 'help against himself' and the therapist says, as it were, 'by my accepting love, I discover in you what you are meant to become'.[19] The discovery is shared by the patient.

Buber held that in a true dialogue both partners must come up against 'the moment of surprise'. The patients are surprised at the development within themselves,[20] and the therapist also goes through 'the moment of surprise', as he experiences a strengthening of his creative power. While the patient's strength grows in the course of the existential treatment, so does the therapist's. While the therapist interprets and serves the patient's existential needs, he gains insight into his own problems and strength to cope with them.

All through the existential treatment, the therapist must preserve the special nature of his therapeutic love which Seguin has defined. He must not allow himself to get entangled in the patient's life, as he could not then provide the help which is required. On the other hand, he must not be indifferent, taking up the attitude of scientific objectivity, of aloofness. This controlled form of involvement, which the therapist has to acquire in his training, is of the utmost importance. The correct relationship with his patients is achieved through continuous self-awareness. In approaching the patient, the therapist approaches himself and meets his own strength and weakness. The therapeutic encounter is a challenge for the therapist and for the patient.

EXISTENTIAL ASSESSMENT

The success of the therapeutic encounter does not only depend on the therapist's moral qualities although these are basic for the treatment. His task requires also medical-clinical judgement. In the discussion of personalistic existential ethics, the limitations of freedom in the neurotic person were stressed and the account of existential psychotherapy must include the existential assessment.

An assessment implies objective estimation. The therapist finds himself here on uncertain ground. The scientist uses the scientific law in his objective approach, but no such general yardstick is available for the existential therapist. His grasp of the patient's personality is intuitive and follows the lines which were discussed in the survey of phenomenological psychiatry. As was pointed out then, this form of understanding does not justify generalizations from one person to the next. There is no fixed pattern in a personal world, for there is continual flux. Therefore the assessment can apply only to the patient's existential resources at a particular moment.

The first factor which determines the chances of successful existential treatment is the patient's attitude, his motivation. Under the influence of scientisms, many people are corrupted and expect the therapist to 'cure' them of their neurosis. Existential psychotherapy relies on a person's determination, on his own efforts, and on the exercise of his freedom.

Through his relationship with the patient, the therapist can judge the patient's sincerity. He has lived with him through the despair of bondage and accepts the genuinness of a note such as the following: 'Life is like living Hell. I have reached the point where I must break through to a better state where I can enjoy – I know not in what way – what remains of the all too fast diminishing period of my life.' He believed also a patient who wrote: 'I cannot live with what I am. . . I have regained the desire to be aware of life and its meaning. I realise now that I have always turned my back on this freedom. . . how can I throw off the old person and adopt a new existence?'

The intention to change is, however, not enough. What also matters is strength. In the choice of the existential methods of treatment, it is vital to assess the patient's power. An LSD treatment, for instance, would be unsuitable and even harmful for one who cannot endure its stirring experience.

Projective tests such as the Rorschach can be applied in order to test the self's resources, but a patient's own drawings can often supply the answer.

The drawing of a patient can illustrate the weakness of a self which cannot gain strength through forceful existential confrontation. This man showed a measure of awareness; looking at the three portraits of himself, he admitted: 'Everything I touch crumbles away' (*Figure 1*).

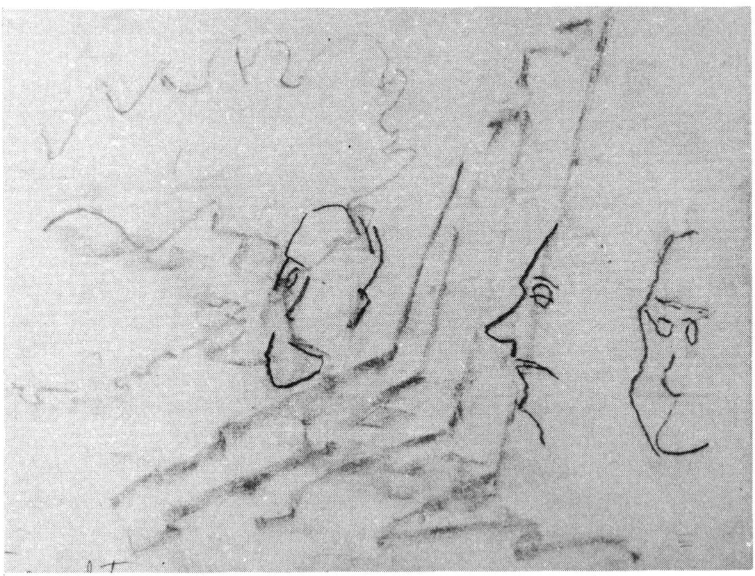

Figure 1

The rising ear of corn, on the other hand, conveys a self which is determined to use its strength, to scatter the forces which have obstructed its growth. This patient responded to existential treatment and gained a good measure of freedom from her neurotic impediment. She accepted the challenge of her life (*Figure 2*).

In contrast to such an effort stands the escape symbolized by the picture of another patient who refused to endure the dark world,

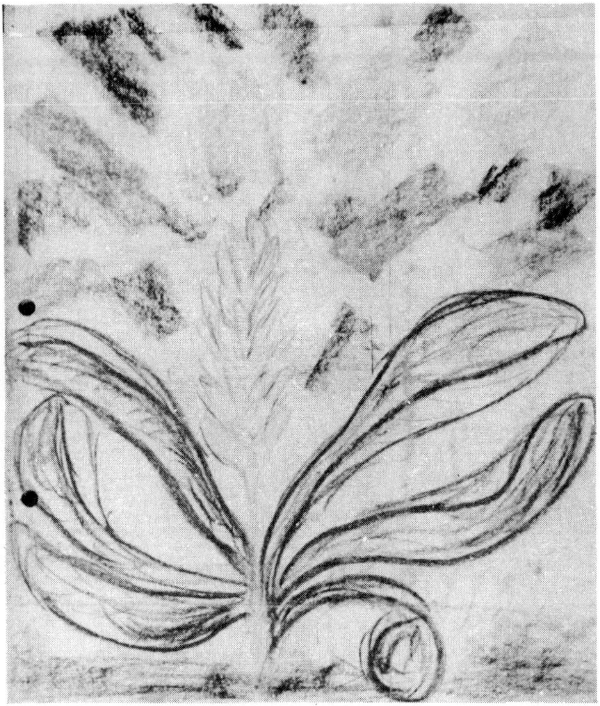

Figure 2

portrayed by the map of Europe below the rainbow. She had taken refuge in a realm high up in the clouds, a world to which drugs gave her access (*Figure 3*).

A series of reveries can reveal a self's poor chances of gaining freedom as it did in the case of a woman who suffered from severe hysterical symptoms; in one treatment, she saw an empty stage and there was nobody in the theatre. She then went out into the street, which was also deserted. Every house was shut up. When she was asked by the therapist: 'What has caused the emptiness and this desolation?' she replied, 'Disappointment, first with mother and father in childhood, later with my husband.' When it was suggested that she should open the shutters, she was unable to do so. In the next treatment, six days later, she was first too afraid to look at the scenery. This fear reminded her of the fear she suffered in childhood. When she found the courage to

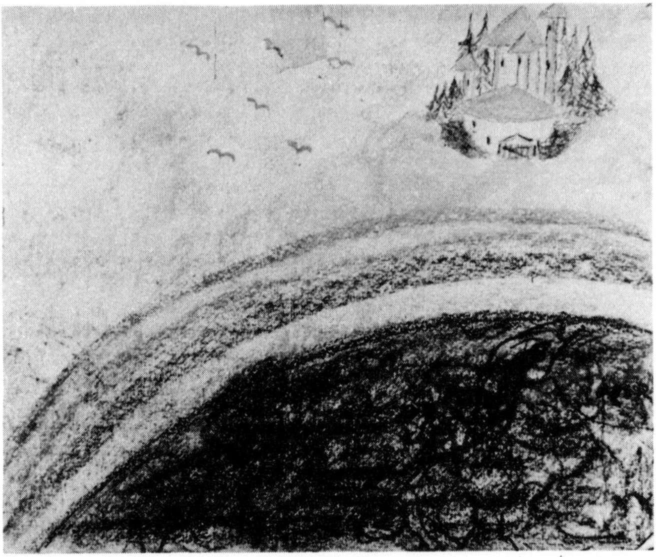

Figure 3

face the stage, there was even greater emptiness than last time. For the street outside the theatre was in ruins, there were no proper houses. She wanted to go home, but she could not find her way.[21]

7

Liberation of the Personal Self

In his existential assessment, the therapist judges the patient's moral intention and moral fibre. The estimation enables him to conduct the treatment. The essence of existential therapy does not, however, consist mainly in the application of the correct measures, but in the patient's own efforts directed at attaining a new existence.

The account of the therapeutic encounter gave an indication of the situation in which both therapist and patient are involved. The latter, in a chaotic state, requires the former's help 'against himself' so that both can discover the patient's potentialities of existence. Although the basic assumption is that he has a conscience and wants to act according to its call, his disturbed mind may not be able to conceive what he is meant to become, his conscience tells him only that his present existence is wrong and intolerable.

Before the new self can be realized, its image must be formed, the image of a person who meets the world in his own rights. In the present chapter, some of the dynamics of the liberation of the patient's personality will be developed and illustrated with accounts from people engaged in this struggle.

EXISTENTIAL AND NON-EXISTENTIAL GUILT

In a medically-orientated personalistic ethic, the liberation of the personality and the discovery of the true personal image depend on the liberation of conscience from its chaotic state. Freedom of conscience was discussed in the exposition of existential ethics and the possibilities of insoluble moral conflicts leading to inevitable guilt were admitted. In such a situation, a person recognizes two opposing duties and he may suffer a breakdown if he is unable to decide between them.

The psychopathology of conscience is complicated by the fact that sick people are not always able to perceive their obligations; in fact, under certain pathological conditions, they may be misled in their moral judgement. The therapist must then protect them against their faulty moral judgements.

An example is the patient who is suffering from depression. Such a person often accuses himself of having ruined his own life and other people's lives. The feelings of guilt have, however, no moral basis and are just a symptom of his disease. They disappear spontaneously when he recovers from this bout of depression. To treat such a patient with the existential approach would be a serious mistake, as it might well increase his symptoms and even lead to suicide.

The case of the neurotic is different from that of a person in psychotic depression. The conscience of the neurotic can be trusted in so far as it perceives correctly that he has failed in his obligations towards himself (and therefore towards others).

Many patients feel safer within their neurotic bondage, to which they have become accustomed and which shields them from taking on the responsibilities of life. By allying themselves with that part of their lives which does not wish to make the effort of liberation, by their lack of motivation, they are guilty, for they are able to recognize their duty. Following this line of thought, Herbert Fingarette defined neurotic guilt as 'the guilt of a person self-blinded, afraid and secretly untrue to his own adult commitment'. As Fingarette has pointed out, a patient's moral judgement may be faulty as 'guilt may be assigned to the wrong source'.[1] It is therefore the task of patient and therapist to discover the true source of the guilt.

A typical example of a faulty assignment of guilt was the case of a single woman who felt guilty when she deviated from her mother's principles, but whose guilt consisted in fact in allowing herself to be dominated by her mother. The situation was expressed in the following note which she sent to her therapist:

> As mother liked nobody, I like nobody. She would say that I should not be friendly with P. or G. because she would make sure that I found something in these women to dislike. Mother's influence overrules my feeling of friendship, does not allow me to get near to them and invite them to my home. I feel guilty at the thought of making friends, no matter who it is, as mother would not approve of them, so I feel I must not approve of them. . . I feel I must not spend money on myself. If I do spend money, especially to improve my home, I feel guilty.

In her treatment the patient was confronted with her real guilt, and she realized that her resistance to mother's wishes and views was – far from being morally wrong – her moral right and duty. Whereas she had felt that she did not deserve to have her own life, feeling guilty when trying to establish her self, she saw that her guilt was, in fact, not to strive for freedom from her mother. As she succeeded in liberating herself from her mother's domination, she lost her feeling of guilt, her self-hatred, and her neurotic symptoms.

Over-dependency on a mother is more the mother's than the daughter's guilt. The daughter is guilty only to the extent to which she fails to break away. This type of guilt can be removed during existential treatment, as the patient gains her freedom.

Some guilt cannot be removed, for instance the guilt of a deed performed in the past. The therapist must try to help such a person to face the guilt and its neurotic consequences which the patient must recognize as a punishment inflicted by conscience. Existential therapy in such a case does not aim at removing the guilt feelings, but at enabling the patient to carry the guilt without increasing it through the manifestation of neurotic symptoms.

The symptoms of neurosis in such a case consisted in severe phobias and in abdominal pain. The guilt was the abortion of an illegitimate pregnancy seventeen years earlier; the patient had suffered from abdominal pain as the interruption of her pregnancy had been followed by peritonitis. The treatment enabled her to face her guilt and benefit from her insight.

The woman who had procured her abortion had no doubt about her guilt. There are, however, cases in which there is doubt, and the existential therapist has to help a patient to clarify the position. An example is a woman who suffered from disabling neurotic symptoms. She felt guilty on account of sexual promiscuity which had started at the age of ten when she was assaulted by a boy of her own age. Behind her parents' back, she had frequent intercourses and had nine lovers before her marriage at the age of twenty-four. Although intercourse was a frightening experience at the beginning, she became 'addicted' to it by the time she was thirteen. She felt guilty at having led a double life, hiding the sexual experiences from her parents (her father was particularly strict).

She argued that she was not guilty when she started her sexual activities, as she had no sexual knowledge then. She partly blamed her parents for the unhappy atmosphere at home and her mother for having failed to enlighten her about sexual matters. On the other hand, she admitted that she was guilty of allowing the habit to grow on her when she realized its significance. Her neurotic illness appeared to her a punishment from God for her sin. This patient faced her moral problem and found relief from her neurotic symptoms.

The therapist may be called upon to assist in the search for a correct moral judgement where a decision of right and wrong cannot be reached. A woman who received treatment for a severe compulsive neurosis felt guilty on account of her promiscuity earlier on in life. Her own mother had been promiscuous and, as this daughter had not been her husband's child, she hated her and called her a 'bastard' when she was only twelve years old. In such a case, the therapist tries to direct the patient's conscience to the duty to make something of her life and not to waste it in further self-punishment.

THE CHALLENGE OF AUTHENTICITY

As was pointed out in the description of personalistic existential ethics, the awareness of the challenge of existence is itself an exercise of a person's freedom. This awareness entails a necessary detachment; for in the words of a patient, 'you can't face something which is so close to you that it is part of you'. She made good use of her freedom which she described as follows: 'Now I can see the old frightened self, it is no more inside me. It seems funny to see life from a frightened child's point of view.' The laughter which accompanied these words signified her freedom from the immersion in her childhood fears.

People have great difficulty in obtaining a new perspective. Such vision was gained by the person who exclaimed: 'I want to find the real me instead of being a machine forced to conform to a pattern which is decided by somebody else.' The realization of the 'real me' in such a case entails a very arduous task. The 'me' was prevented from coming into being through a suppressive upbringing and the 'machine' self was the result of the inhibition of her authenticity.

The therapist has to choose the right moment to face the patient with his need to change, and such a confrontation can be a painful shock, as the following outburst testifies:

> You said I wasn't a proper person. At the time you said it, it didn't seem to affect me very much, but as soon as I left you, I was suddenly overwhelmed by the full meaning of your words. I was deeply shocked at realizing that I was not a proper person, because, this being so, I have absolutely nothing to commend me. I am a total loss. I felt this, and I wanted to die. You see, I completely accepted your remark. In your opinion, I wasn't a proper person, and then I felt the truth of this remark. The shock of this truth was so severe, as I had been quite unaware of it.

The letter was discussed during the next session. The patient admitted that she had intended to make the therapist feel guilty for having given her such a painful experience. She recognized the fact that she had to blame somebody. But she overcame this resentment and benefited from the experience.

To achieve authenticity, the patient has to become aware of his inauthenticity and has to investigate his subjective world, so that he can recognize his challenge. The following dream of a single woman of forty-four illustrates her predicament: 'In front of me I saw a closed window. I knew I must open it, otherwise I would not get any air to breathe. So I tried to pull the top half open, which I managed to do after a hard struggle. But, to my horror, I saw then that the window was right against a brick wall, so that no air could get into the room.'

The same patient described in a note to her therapist in what sense her inner world was stifling: 'I am so completely smothered and surrounded by fear: fear of things, of people, of sensations, of myself and of my own reactions and feelings.' The therapist gave her insight into one specific fear during a reverie treatment. She referred to this discovery when she wrote to him after the session: 'I feel so ashamed at having to admit in the reverie today that I feel such awful fear even with you. It seems terrible after all these years of treatment, but there was no escaping the fact which I had refused to admit even to myself.'

An LSD treatment enabled her to experience her longing for freedom which was manifest in the following hallucination:

> I was at the sea standing on a beach alone, with a terrific longing to be free. I wanted to take my clothes off to be completely free and wanted this not to matter. I knew everybody else did this, and I was the only person who was held tightly back.

In a dream, this inhibited woman found herself changing her attitude towards her body and this change was symbolized as follows:

> I arrived at the hospital for my appointment. I could not get into the cloakroom where I had to change my clothes before I saw the doctor. After a long wait, I found myself changing in another room, a woman fastened my bra, and I then put on a pair of knickers and went into the room for my appointment.

She had realized that her tension was due to her fear of losing control over herself.

> I am so frightened of losing my hold. . . of not being in perfect control, of speaking without first thinking of the effect of my words, of my words just coming out of my mouth, no matter what they might be – and yet, part of me longs so desperately to do this.

Her fear was thus of her own responses and of the reactions from others, and she saw that her self was deprived of authenticity by her world of tight emotional control. To gain the freedom of her feelings, she said, was 'essential if I am to become completely human'.

The tight control was also directed against her body. In the LSD experience, her whole body felt dead when she touched it. She could not use the word breasts in speaking or writing. On hearing anyone else even mentioning this word, she felt 'extremely insecure and terribly frightened, as if something dreadful will happen to me, even if I hear the word spoken, some sort of punishment. . . So far as I was concerned bodies did not exist, not even my own. It never entered my head to touch another person, not even a child. I am even afraid of my own body, afraid to realize that it is something alive and afraid to touch and to feel it.' She added that she had never recognized this fear before. The awareness was thus gained through the existential treatment.

The possession of an adult body can be a serious challenge to the self of an immature person. A married woman of thirty-five, the mother of three children, admitted to her therapist that she was astonished at having an adult body. Patients discover these fears under existential treatment, and such discovery is essential if they are to face their fear and overcome it.

Facing the sexual instinct is part of the challenge presented by the body. The dream of a homosexual man relates how he accepted nakedness, but not his sexuality, which he omitted in the characters of the following dream: 'It began to get very hot. I decided to take my clothes off. . . I saw a negro and two coloured children. They were completely naked, and I was surprised that they had no sex organs.'

A denial of sexuality can bring about many neurotic disturbances. The patient who is frightened of facing his or her sexuality does not necessarily realize the connection between his symptoms and his fears. Existential therapy can bring about such realization. An LSD session brought this liberating insight to a girl whose life had been crippled by neurotic symptoms the sexual significance of which she had not grasped before. Through the treatment she achieved complete freedom from her illness.

Those who cannot overcome their barriers often experience anger, jealousy of more fortunate people, resentment, and other destructive emotions. To admit to the violence of anger can be necessary for overcoming it. A patient who made the world responsible for her emotional blockage, described her violent phantasies as follows:

> It is so awful, I would just love to hit somebody tonight, to have others at my mercy, instead of being at theirs. I would love to hurt them as they have hurt me, and are still hurting me. To make them suffer as they have made me suffer, to let them have a taste of their own medicine, and to see how they liked it. Nothing, just nothing could be too hurtful to do to them over and over again, until they are squashed and useless, and never able to rise again –

not to actually kill them, because if they were killed, they would not feel pain and despair, and they must be made to feel it, as they have made me feel it. I would love to deprive them of everything they want and hope for in every way, I would ruin their lives and make certain that everybody ignored them and trampled on them, squashing them to nothing.

This same patient expressed her flaming anger in a picture, the black outer part of which denotes her depression. The pale area which surrounds the flame indicates, however, that the world beyond can appear more peaceful (*Figure 4*).

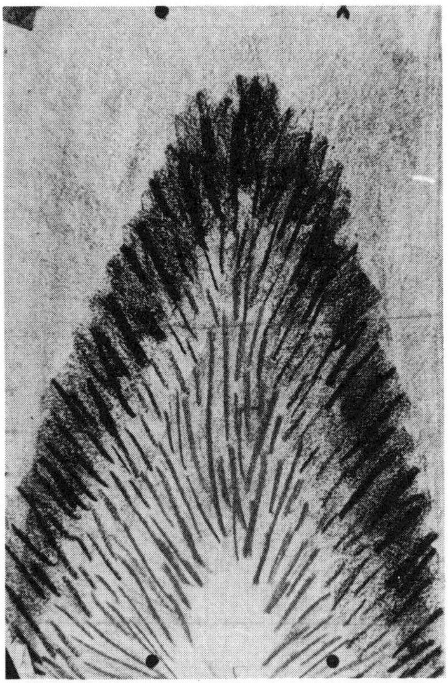

Figure 4

Although it is necessary to allow the self to express its protest against its bondage and although, in this patient's case, it was an achievement to give vent to her anger in words and in a drawing, the existential therapist does not hold that aggressiveness is a primary instinct which has to be liberated. To him, aggressiveness is a destructive reaction to a situation in which the self finds itself frustrated. By facing the situation and the anger which it causes, the patient can free himself from the bondage of his resentment.

An outburst of uncontrolled rage must be distinguished from a controlled angry insistence on one's rights. A patient who had been afraid to assert herself because of fear of others found under existential treatment the courage to protest to her employer against having been given too much work. Such protest is a positive achievement and makes the person more authentic; the anger which is expressed in this manner is channelled into constructive ways and is not destructive, as is an outburst of uncontrolled rage.

The force of anger can stimulate the self's awareness. A woman of fifty-three who had failed to have good relationships with her husbands in two marriages felt the sting of jealousy when she thought of her daughter's happy marriage. This patient recognized the annoyance as directed at her own failure. The insight led to a better relationship with her daughter and to a feeling of greater authenticity.

FACING THE ORIGIN OF INAUTHENTICITY

Meeting the challenge of inauthenticity involves facing its origin. When discussing existential guilt, we saw that people have to go back into their past and have to realize where their inauthenticity started.

The weak self is the self of childhood. In the treatment the neurotic is helped to overcome his fears and to trace his present insecurity to the first years of his life. By returning the patient to his early memories, the existential therapist does not 'regress' him to the state of helpless infancy. The purpose of the treatment is to enable him to experience his present potential strength of adulthood in contrast to his childhood weakness which he has carried with him.

The existential therapist's attitude towards regression follows from his basic assumption of human freedom. He differs fundamentally from the attitude of the deterministically-minded analyst who follows D. W. Winnicott's view on therapeutic regression. This author aimed at taking an adult patient back to the infantile state of development in which the therapist fulfils the role of the mother in order to 'give the patient a last chance to grow a real self'.[2] In Winnicott's view, an adult is unable to liberate himself from his neurotic bondage, as he is fully determined by his libidinal object relationships.

People are frequently quite unaware of the process which blocks their potentialities and of the source of their bondage. The existential therapist has to help them to gain the 'genetic understanding' which was described in the section on phenomenological psychiatry, so that they can obtain insight into the development of their attitudes and of the influences which were responsible for them. As Jaspers has pointed out, 'this mode of self-understanding becomes a factor in [a person's] psychic development'.[3]

People are afraid to look back because they find themselves in conflict with the loyalities of their past and with the values which they had accepted. The more thorough their examination of their lives, the more reasons do they find for distrusting their cherished beliefs. Such a journey of discovery involves facing the truth that so much life has been wasted, and that the people on whom they depended, such as parents and teachers, were causes of their unhappy state. As the patient, encouraged and supported by the therapist, appreciates the significance of his former experiences, he gains strength and determination to achieve the necessary insight. We shall now trace some of these tragedies.

The following is an account of a girl's dehumanization perpetrated by parents and teachers:

> When I was about four years old, I wanted someone to play with me. I was told that I should be content to play by myself with all the lovely toys which I had been given and I should not want anything or anybody else. Being unable to convey my feelings, I just remained dumb and did not answer – feeling a terrible pain, feeling there must be something wrong with me. At school I never looked at the nuns as human beings, the words 'human being' never entered my mind.
>
> Boys just did not exist in my mind, now I realize I never thought of them as human beings, as I never thought of myself as one. They were some kind of object with which one must be very careful and keep at a distance, or else terrible things happened. The thought that boys were in any way different from girls was completely outside my knowledge, as I grew up.

It is not surprising that this patient, an only child, withdrew into a world of phantasy and became ill.

Her father was very domineering, he terrified her and her mother. In one of her dreams, his suppressive influence was symbolized: he was lying across her legs, thus immobilizing her.

Mother's influence in preventing her from becoming a person was perhaps even greater than father's although the patient needed great courage to admit this truth. Mother had been unable to tolerate her daughter's sexual maturity. She had forced her to wear tight clothes around her chest for years to hide her developing breasts which were 'squashed'. The patient recalled this experience as 'something I shall never forget; it was like squashing the life out of me. The pain in my chest was dreadful when I undressed at night. I just had to stick it and suffer in silence. I feel this has scarred me for life.

The girl was completely in her mother's power, as the following dream pointed out to her:

> I entered a cinema and could see my mother sitting in one of the centre rows. There were vacant seats, one next to my mother. I knew I must not and could not sit down without having been given permission. I waited for mother's signal in vain and was left standing in the gangway with no chance to sit down in comfort like all the other people.

Her mother's attitude became obvious to her through a dream in which she found herself on the way to America, which stood in her mind for the country of freedom; she was with her mother, who had hidden her flight ticket so that she missed the aeroplane.

This patient reported the following progress which was greatly helped by LSD: 'I feel I achieved a lot. I feel far more wide awake, as if my eyes had been opened, so that I look down on things, that I am on top of them instead of being underneath them.'

A mother's part in depriving a daughter from achieving authenticity can be much less obvious than it was in this last example. A single woman of thirty-five had been brought up by a most 'devoted' mother who had impressed on her children her strict Christian outlook. With the aid of LSD, this patient saw clearly that her mother had in fact prevented her from making a life of her own, that she had made all her family feel guilty when they wanted to enjoy themselves, and had used religion as a weapon against them. The patient's anger against her mother, the first reaction to her insight, was overcome, and she managed to forge ahead without being under mother's domination and without hating her.

A sensitive child can be frightened by the roughness of life. A married woman of twenty-seven who suffered from a number of phobias which crippled her life could not account for her fears. When questioned about her parents she described them as kind people who had brought her up with affection and understanding.

Under the influence of LSD she relived scenes which had terrified her as a child and which had been suppressed into her unconscious: her father had struck her as a cruel man, he had snared rabbits, had killed a cat which she had loved, and had kicked the dog so that he had had to be destroyed. She also remembered the death of a horse and of a cockrel who had suffered a horrible end. Because of these terrifying experiences, she had refused to meet the world.

This patient's treatment was successful. She found fulfilment in her marriage and became a person in her own right, standing up to her husband and to his mother.

As long as a mother conveys to her child some kind of love, even if it is a possessive love, the child can develop, although the development is badly damaged if the love is selfish. But if a child feels completely rejected by his mother, he is stunted emotionally. Such a person withdraws into a world of unreality and cuts himself off from the real world which has become unbearable to him. He is not aware of the origin of his imprisonment, however, as it would be too painful to face the existential trauma. Existential psychotherapy aims at lifting such an experience into consciousness.

If the patient is judged fit for confrontation with his early traumatic experience, the therapist can use LSD or other drugs to make him aware of the origin of his neurosis. This method was used in the case of a married man of twenty-four. The patient was first admitted into hospital at the age of eighteen when he gave a history of depression with bouts of crying. The provisional diagnosis was schizophrenia, but the final diagnosis was personality disorder. He stayed in the hospital for one year, worked for the next three years, then was re-admitted because he could not work. He did not join in group discussions or occupational therapy, remaining anxious, depressed, and embarrassed. After three months, he was discharged and attended as an out-patient, but failed to respond to treatment and remained unwilling to attempt any work.

Various psychological tests indicated an inability to express his feelings, a state of confusion, and a weakness of his self. The psychologist considered the use of LSD to be risky, as the self did not appear strong enough for this form of treatment. During the first nine months of the existential treatment, drugs were not given. Discussions confirmed the impression gained by the former therapist that this patient was frightened of life. A dream was significant: he first tried to swim across a river, but gave up his attempt, as it would not be safe.

As no progress was made and as the therapist, differing from the psychologist, judged the patient fit for LSD experiences, LSD, combined with methylamphetamine and methylphenidate, was given with close support from the therapist. The patient now re-lived his early childhood, he felt abandoned by his parents and frightened, especially during air raids. In the eleventh LSD session he went through the experience which, he was convinced, had crippled his life: when he was three years old, his mother had tried to suffocate him.

The therapist could not check up on the truth of this allegation; there was no doubt that the mother had neglected her children, but the patient may have had a phantasy of this murderous attempt upon him. The important thing was not to find out what was objectively true, but what was true subjectively, to obtain a true picture of his world which he had to face with the therapist's help. The patient realized that his mother's rejection had prevented him from trusting other people and had caused him to hide himself away from the world. He felt too insecure to undertake the work expected of a man. He could not bear to return to the world of childhood desolation except when freed from the most acute anxiety through injections of amylobarbitone and methylamphetamine. With protection from these drugs he found the courage to face the origin of his inauthenticity.

A child's faith in his mother may be shattered by the feeling that he owes her special thanks, that it is up to him to make her happy. Such a situation is more serious if the child has been adopted, as his trust was shaken when he was told that his real mother had given him away. A young man of eighteen traced his inability to face people to the feelings with which he grew up as an adopted child. He told his therapist that he was expected to give his adopted parents happiness in return for their having adopted him. 'I must never upset them in any way; for if I did, they would say that I had never loved them.' He experienced their expectation of love as emotional blackmail. He could not be spontaneous and had to 'put on an act of liking them'. As he had gained insight into the origin of his emotional breakdown, he was able to explain to his therapist and to himself:

> I broke down when the act became too great an emotional strain.
> I felt afraid that they could see that I was pretending to love them.
> I felt that they were trying to catch me out and were thus against me.

This patient realized that a life of pretence is wrong and he tried to be sincere. He thus grasped the conflict with which he had grown up:

> Half my mind was saying, 'I must put on an act', and the other half told me not to do it. Being unable to stop the acting, I turned against myself. As I could not approve of myself, I thought that other people did not approve of me either. With this suspicion in my mind, I could not trust people.

He then described how he became estranged from the world:

> I began to find faults with people, telling myself that they were no good. But I did not want them to know my opinion of them, so I tried to cover it up. . . I feared, however, that they would find out and I was afraid of the result of this discovery.

This young man saw the possibility of his freedom when he wrote: 'To overcome my problem, I must realize that I have no obligation to make people happy.'

THE STRUGGLE FOR THE REALIZATION OF AUTHENTICITY

The act of awareness constitutes one facet of freedom. It opens up vistas of new existence. In the exposition of personalistic existential ethics Karl Jaspers' observations threw light on the significance of awareness which, we learnt, can enable a person to distinguish himself from others. Many people lack the confirmation which comes with consciousness of individuality. We were assured by Jaspers that the person who is aware of himself is also aware of his value. This experience is decisive for those who are lacking in a feeling of personal worth and dignity. Furthermore, awareness meets the human need for making sense of the experiences which man gathers: it provides 'meaningful connections'.[4]

The healing effect of awareness was traced to 'a release from the obscure bondage of the undifferentiated, from the given thus-ness of the self (Sosein), from the power of uncritically accepted symbols and from the absolute reality of the objective world. . . It is a relief that at last I know what up to then I have only felt'.[5]

Awareness of the inauthenticity of one's existence and of the origin and development of this inauthenticity does not by itself lead to a more authentic existence. Jaspers is too optimistic when he holds that 'if I know what happens to me, I have taken the first step to freedom in contrast to being blindly overpowered';[6] for the weak person may not be able to act in accordance with the insight of his awareness.

For awareness to be liberating, it must lead to a new orientation within the world of experience which must, in turn, express itself in the 'outer world' as an ability to cope with life situations. The person who has gained this freedom realizes his strength and his limitations and does not waste his life in resentment and destructiveness.

'Inner' experience is essential for gaining freedom 'outside'. One patient expressed this necessity when she said: 'Not experiencing in phantasy would deprive me of the certainty that there are possibilities deep inside me, waiting to be released.' The same patient distinguished between various depths of experience which she had under LSD:

> In LSD treatments I have found that the more deeply I experience something, the more am I able to work through the experience and get the better of it. The superficial experience without LSD is a cooled-off experience which does not enable me to sense what lies deeply buried in me. I might talk about my troubles without feeling the full emotional impact and might transfer the experience to the intellectual level, missing the core of my situation and the chance of facing it.

The following outcry of a girl who had traced her neurosis to a lack of maternal love, illustrates the futility of mere awareness, as the patient felt too weak to undertake the struggle for an authentic existence:

> There is love between my mother and her other children, that gives them the strength to live and to move on, while I am rooted

in fear and bitterness. I can't even rise from my bed, can't get the strength to go to work, go out into the world, not even to the shops. Mother's love is their food, primal food. That is what I must get before I can feed my flesh and blood. I have cried for this love in vain, my chest aches with melancholia. My hope is getting fainter and fainter. Instead, there is a load of vile, fiendish feelings and utterances, love is turning into hate.

To win the struggle for authenticity, a person has to experience his strength and his potentialities. Many patients are greatly helped if they see in dreams or reveries two selves, one weak and sick, and the other strong and healthy. With encouragement from the therapist the strong self carries out the struggle for authenticity and the patient can transfer his victory from the world of fantasy to the world of reality, meeting his life situations with the strength which he has gained in the treatment. Such battles are often prolonged and the victory of the strong self may hang in the balance for a long time.

A dream of a nineteen-year old youth illustrates a critical phase in his bid for freedom: he first saw himself as a cripple, then he became a normal person, but collapsed and found himself dragged down by his parents and his uncle.

A woman aged thirty-nine, who suffered from severe hysterical depression, saw herself in a reverie as two selves, one which was weak, the other appeared to be strong, but her strength was not real, only put on, a 'bravado', false self. This patient experienced her struggle in another reverie by finding herself faced by a choice between two roads, one leading to a mental hospital, the other to life. She realized the significance of both. She did not want to be confined to the hospital, but she was frightened to take the road to freedom, as she did not feel strong enough to face life. There was a gate in front of the second road, the space in front of the gate was dark, but beyond the gate she saw the light of freedom. In spite of this vision, she could not summon the strength to open the gate.

Another patient who had neglected many possibilities of a more authentic existence found herself in a dream trying to open locked doors which led to a more fulfilled life; the struggle which she had with the locks represented her struggle for authenticity.

The challenge of authenticity involves the outgrowing of childish exhibitions of temper. In order to let a man of twenty-four cope with his childhood violence, the therapist asked him to take on the role of the (adult) producer in a reverie in which he was playing out temper tantrums as a child. In this scene, the patient saw himself as a boy of eight, getting furious because his toy train would not run properly. His wife (who had to put up with his tempers) was also on the stage and laughed at his immature behaviour. He, as a child, burst into tears. Then, as the adult producer, he pointed out to the child that he had to grow up. This man made good progress towards authenticity through the insight which he had gained in the struggles within his world of fantasy and through his determination to apply these insights to the life in his world of reality.

The division into an immature, childish self belonging to the past, and a mature, adult self belonging to the present and the future may not be appropriate. There are patients whose potential adult selves are held back by a deed committed in the past and who have to return to this time of their lives in order to gain the freedom of an authentic existence. The deed may have caused a moral conflict and the guilt feelings may have produced incapacitating neurotic symptoms; while the existential therapist does not deny the existence of guilt, he must help his patient to cope with guilt feelings and to gain freedom.

The example of existential guilt which was quoted before was the case of a woman who had procured an abortion years before the beginning of her existential treatment. Her abdominal pain represented the pain which she suffered at that time and, in addition, she complained of a choking feeling in her throat. A reverie symbolized her guilty deed and gave her insight into the significance of her symptoms: on the stage, she saw a cat eating its kitten and then spitting it out. In the discussion, she associated the cat's destruction of its young with her own attack upon her unborn child, and the cat's regurgitation of the kitten with her own painful throat where her deed had 'stuck'. This explanation helped her to bear her guilt and to realize her potentialities; she was relieved of her neurotic incapacity.

Therapist and patient rejoice over the gain of authentic freedom, over the victory won in the existential struggle. Unfortunately, they cannot expect the victory to be final. They have to face the tragic truth that a man may be caught again by the forces which restricted him in the past. His freedom then consists in defying these forces to the best of his ability rather than giving in to them. There is consolation in the fact that the effort needed for the continuation of the battle is not wasted and that one's strength can increase through having braved the loss of freedom and not having evaded the 'antinomic situation', as Karl Jaspers has called it.[7]

8

Liberation of Transcendence

The existential therapist helps the patient in his struggle for authenticity, for his personal selfhood, in his need for self-assurance so that he can stand up for himself and meet the world.

Existential ethics affirms the freedom which is won when man transcends himself. As has already been pointed out, transcendence is not reserved for the saint and the mystic, but is essential for all men so that they can face life and death.[1] The existential therapist must therefore help his patients to gain certainty of transcendence. One patient described the discovery of her self-transcendence, gained through having attended a therapeutic social club, in the following note:

> Something had been getting in the way between me and the worth-while part – and this "something", I believe now, was my own self. *I* did not think the treatment was doing *me* any good, *I* did not like mixing with strangers, *I* wanted to choose the people I mixed with, *I* was not always interested in what was going on, *I* was decidedly frightened of hospitals, noise, crowds, *I* did not think anyone there liked me, – in fact, I, ME and MYSELF were getting thoroughly in the way, and although I made a great effort to join in and to *appear* co-operative and sociable, it was not until I *became* co-operative and sociable, and consequently less frightened and worried, that any real benefit was derived.

TRANSCENDENCE IN COMMUNICATION

Once the I has got out of the way, a person may be ready to communicate, to meet the Thou and to have the transcendental experience which he requires to cope with life. Communication presents a problem for the neurotic and it is necessary to investigate the difficulties which prevent patients from communicating freely and to examine the relevant pathology.

There are degrees of communication. Psychiatrists know that many withdrawn schizophrenics communicate without words, that they satisfy their needs for human contact by sitting silently in the consulting room or in places where their fellow patients gather. Although these patients live in a private world, shut off from the rest of humanity, they are not self-sufficient, but suffer from the loneliness of their isolation.

The neurotic is less isolated than the psychotic, as his illness leaves more room for communion than a psychosis. But the neurotic is self-centred, absorbed in his suffering and thus not freely available for his fellow human being. Existential psychotherapy makes him aware of his need for communication and helps him to express his friendly feelings towards others.

A single, very lonely woman experienced her desire for a human relationship in an LSD treatment and told her psychiatrist afterwards: 'I wanted to hug and love something – just anything that would accept my love. During the treatment, I was too afraid to tell you this and to think about it, and, in any case, I did not know how to tell you.'

For the person who is sure of himself, relationships are easy. To him, there is no pain or fear in losing himself, in giving himself to the other, but the patient who is unsure of himself may experience severe anxiety in such situations. The following note from a woman patient illustrates this restriction of freedom:

> I lose myself in the other. When I get involved in a conversation with one of my colleagues, I am unaware of myself at the time of speaking, but when I withdraw from them, something from them has influenced me so that the original me has become unidentifiable to me. I then do not know who I am and cannot find myself. I feel all at sea, anchorless and in pieces.

The patient considered the following explanation for her disintegration: 'Is it that, deep down, I feel insecure because I revealed something of myself which up to then I had kept to myself?' She then came to the conclusion that she was afraid of others knowing her, but she admitted she did not know the reason for this fear.

The reason why people are afraid of others, of being known by them, is often their feeling of unworthiness. The following poem, written by a lonely woman who had spent her childhood in an orphanage and many years of her life in a mental hospital, expressed her lack of security, her feeling of unfitness for human society, and her conviction that the others were far superior to her.

What Is ME AND WHO ARE THEY?

She is she,
He is he,
They are they,
But please tell me
What is me?

Me is all troubled,
Me is all muddled,
Me is all sad,
Me is quite mad.

Me can't remember,
Me can't forget,
Me is just soppy,
Me is quite wet.

Me is a dope,
A dope without hope,
Me is a clot,
A dirty great blot.

They are the ones who do everything one can't do,
They are the ones who do everything one didn't do,
They are the ones who do what they should do,
They are never the ones who do what they shouldn't do.

The therapist frequently recognizes in what way a patient makes himself unacceptable to his fellow human beings. The patient is usually quite unaware of the reason for his unpopularity, but the treatment can enlighten him.

For example, a man who had put people off by inconsiderate behaviour, but who had been quite oblivious of the effects of his actions on others, felt moved by the following dream:

> I am travelling in an underground train with a lot of luggage [which travellers in the underground are not expected to bring with them]. When I arrive at my destination, I get into a panic, as there is not enough time to collect all my luggage and leave the train. I throw several pieces on the platform and hold my hand between the open doors, hoping the guard will take notice and keep the train waiting. But he does not notice and the doors close while I am still in the train with the rest of my luggage.

This patient was treated in a group which gave him the opportunity for the degree of communication of which he was capable. Through comments from the members of the group, on the above dream, he gained insight into his social handicap.

Group therapy is not suitable for those who can relate to the therapist only in individual treatment. The need for such an exclusive communication was expressed in the following note addressed by a woman patient to her therapist:

> I only feel alright when I am imagining talking to you about things that have happened or things I have done or seen. I like to shut myself away in my own room where I am entirely alone and where it is quiet, to sit there and to tell you all these things. When I mix with other people, their talk just bounces back on me; if I talk to them my words sound far away and they also bounce back as though no one had received them. When I sit with other patients, I see myself sitting with them, but it feels that it is not myself who is sitting there. It is very uncanny, like seeing oneself in a mirror or in a film.
>
> My room is like a tomb with just you and me talking in it and I don't want anyone to intrude or unlock it.
>
> I feel as if some terrific power is beginning to catch hold of me. I don't know what to do about it, I can't keep the door locked any more, it is surely beginning to open. The key was in the hands of someone I loved very dearly and deeply, someone who broke my heart. Why is he trying to unlock the tomb?
>
> I buried the ghost of this person a long time ago with myself. I thought I had thrown the key away, but you have picked it up.
>
> I haven't the strength to come out after all these years, and yet I am in your power which is stronger than mine, and I am so frightened.

The person who had the key originally was her father with whom the patient lost touch when she was sent to an orphanage in her early childhood. Had this patient transferred her love from her father to her therapist? Had the existential therapist accepted the Freudian concept of the transference? The answer to both questions is no.

As O. Fenichel has explained, the psycho-analytical interpretation involves two aspects of the transference phenomenon. Firstly, it is 'considered as a form of resistance'. In other words, the Freudian assumes that 'the patient defends himself against remembering and discussing his infantile conflicts by reliving them',[2] and evades this task by forming a relationship of love or hatred with the therapist instead.

The existentialist agrees that it may be painful for the patient to relive the infantile relationships, but he denies that a relationship with the therapist is an escape from such pain; for the existentialist, each communication between people is personal, unique and genuine, whereas to the psychoanalyst it is just a libidinal discharge. This difference is revealed by Fenichel's second point: Transference actions are to him substitutions for original connections and hence distortions. Because of this fault, 'the discharge thus attained is necessarily insufficient'.[3]

The existentialist agrees in this case with Rollo May who has pointed out that 'what really happens is not that the neurotic patient "transfers" feelings he had toward mother or father to wife or therapist. Rather, the neurotic is one who in certain areas never developed beyond the limited and restricted forms of experience characteristic of the infant'. Therefore 'the concept of transference in the sense of a displacement of detachable feelings from one object to another [is] unnecessary',[4] and the patient who was locked in the tomb of her childhood isolation must be encouraged through the new relationship with her therapist to free herself by facing her anxiety and by employing her adult strength in her present communication. The existential therapist conceives of the I-Thou relationships with his patients as encounters and not as libidinal transactions.

The aim of the treatment must, of course, be to help the patient to open up to other people and not to be entirely dependent on his therapist. This goal must be conveyed to the patient in the treatment and the relationship between patient and therapist must be faced, but not analysed in the Freudian sense as a revival of childhood relationships.

The existential therapist confronts his patients with the challenges presented by their personal relationships, with father, mother, child, husband, wife, and others. The failure to establish a good relationship may date back to early childhood. In fact, a mother or father may have died, but the person is still suffering from the unresolved conflict with the parent. The treatment attempts to resolve such a conflict.

The following reverie indicated the turning point in a woman's unhappy relationship with her husband and the adoption of a new attitude towards him: she found herself walking through a long tunnel, the husband was waiting at the other end. She realized that he looked uncertain, so she met him and gave him confidence.

The freedom of personal communication is the freedom from self-centredness and the awareness of the fellow human being in his needs. For the transcendence of communication to be realized, the I which is concerned only about itself has to get out of the way. Once the way is clear, communication occurs spontaneously, without effort.

A very lonely and withdrawn, shy woman experienced this temporary liberation from her isolation when, during a visit to a hospital ward, she noticed a woman patient having difficulty drying her hair with an electric dryer. The visitor went to her help and dried her hair for her. This form of silent communication was a unique achievement, a meeting with her transcendence. She recognized its significance when she wrote: 'I surprised myself doing something for another person which I am quite certain I would never have been able to do before my LSD treatment. I just could not stop myself.'

In an unselfish communication, in an I-Thou relationship, each personal self gives way to the other, but finds itself re-established through confirmation by the other. In such a communion, a person is assured of his transcendence and is for the time being relieved of the symptoms arising from the noogenic neurosis. Existential therapy aims at this liberation.

TRANSCENDENCE IN CREATIVENESS

Man does not only transcend himself in the relationship with the fellow human beings, he does so also in creative activities. In both cases he forgets his personal self. A small child is lost in his game, an adult in an absorbing task, but the neurotic is held back by his concern about himself. He is selfconscious, and is thus barred from his creativeness.

Denigration on the self in childhood or adolescence can bring about a crippling of a creative personality. A single young woman who had often been told by her mother that she was a complete failure could not fulfil the promise of her artistic talents and complete her course at an art school. She was stopped by fear of destructive criticism from her teachers, who in her imagination carried on mother's part and also by the fear of competition with her fellow students. During existential treatment she realized the nature of her handicap and gradually overcame it.

Another patient, a married man, was unable to finish his architecture course because he could not design buildings and therefore could not meet the creative demands of his profession; he was not even able to build a sand castle when playing with his young children. With treatment, he recognized not only his fear of losing himself in creative activities, but also the forces which held him back: his resentment against his mother's ambition, echoed by his wife, and fear of facing the possibility of failure when sitting for the final examination. In addition, he realized that he was afraid of the responsibilities which he would have to shoulder as a qualified architect. He traced his lack of confidence back to his childhood when he was evacuated during the war and felt scared. In an LSD session, he experienced his inability to let himself go, as he had been deprived of the security of maternal love which allows a child freedom of creativeness.

Very severe emotional insecurity in early childhood caused another patient, a trained motor mechanic, such inhibition of his creative abilities that he could not face working on motor cars. It was significant that he could at times dismantle an engine without much difficulty, but the re-assembling of parts, the constructive and creative side of his work, caused him unbearable anxiety. He became aware of the same kind of difficulty when helping his wife in the kitchen; he could wash up dishes for her, but he could not put the clean dishes into the cupboard, could not create 'a pattern'.

A further patient, a hairdresser, was unsuccessful in giving a customer's hair the final shape. Like the motor mechanic, he discovered that he was held back by the fear of the unknown, the new. A painter admitted that he had used only about five per cent of his time for productive work, the rest of the time he put off working to 'some future date which never came'. He had escaped by drinking and going abroad. Before his treatment, he had not recognized 'the pattern of repeated failure' and had considered himself just 'somewhat eccentric, but quite normal otherwise'. He said: 'I was quite unaware of the fact that I was wasting my life.' This new awareness, he felt, had made the escapes impossible. He admitted to his therapist: 'No retreat is now open to me. I am face to face with my fear of life, which was carefully covered up before.' As the result of this insight, there was a liberation of his artistic creativeness

TRANSCENDENCE IN DECISION

When giving himself to creative work or to a fellow human being, man surrenders his personal self, gaining fulfilment and confirmation of his transcendence. In the act of decision, however, man experiences transcendence without any assurance of compensation. When making a choice, he takes a risk and gives up the certainty of the position which he had held. By choosing one thing in favour of another, he renounces the thing which he has rejected; man requires, therefore, strength and courage for the leap of decision.

In the exposition of personal existential ethics, freedom of the decision has already been discussed. It is now necessary to supply some details of existential psychotherapy to illustrate the psychopathology connected with this form of transcendence.

The anguish which man faces in the moment of commitment has already been evidenced by Sartrian characters who fail to make the necessary choices. They are the archetype of the neurotic faithless person who procrastinates endlessly, who avoids saying yes or no, who allows loopholes and escapes in all his actions, revokes his decisions immediately after having made them, and avoids making an absolute choice.

Many neurotics make excellent resolutions which, however, are not carried out; therefore they fail to gain the freedom of their authenticity and the experience of their transcendence.

In an age in which people are insured against all sorts of risks, the individual is not encouraged to make daring decisions. The following dream of a patient illustrates the dilemma of irresolution: 'I want to swim in a pool, but I am warned not to do so, as there is a dangerous current. So I hesitate, as I cannot see where the current is going to.' It is a common excuse when avoiding a vital decision that one is not in the right mood, that one feels too depressed at the time and has to wait for the strength and courage of a more optimistic frame of mind. Through existential therapy, a patient recognized that these moods were not just fateful, but that he had some freedom in their making. He reported this discovery in the following note:

> I swing, like a pendulum, between the states of optimism when I feel full of courage, and pessimism, when I am depressed. I used to describe these phases as 'having the current turned on or off'. I now realize that it is *I* who turn it on and off. LSD has made me aware of this situation for the first time.

He was strong enough to carry out the decision to keep the 'current' on.

Another patient realized in an LSD session that an unconscious decision had ruined his life and needed to be revoked:

> I must stop despising myself. If a man decides 'I am contemptible', then all apparent evidence showing the contrary is dismissed by him. The illusion of being contemptible becomes more important than the facts concerning his intrinsic worth. If one despises oneself, then obviously one assumes that others despise one, and love and trust cannot be built on despisal.

Claustrophobia and agarophobia can express a person's fear of making decisions. These symptoms keep him from entering into a place from which he cannot get out, such as an underground train when it is in motion. They stop him from leaving the safe home and venturing into the open. The following example illustrates such fear.

The patient was a man of thirty-four whose work entailed travelling long distances. He could not undertake such journeys, as he often felt giddy and experienced sudden panics. During the treatment he realized that he had allowed himself to be held back by a close relationship with his mother. He found the courage to carry out the decision to make himself independent of her when, under LSD, he re-lived a scene which had occurred, in his school life; after he had broken down and cried, an older boy said, 'Be a man!' He discovered that he had to choose manliness now and achieved freedom from his mother and from his symptom.

TRANSCENDENCE IN FACING THE INEVITABLE

By daring to make a decision, by getting absorbed in creative activities, and by relating himself to the other, man transcends himself and at the same time is confirmed in his personal authenticity. He thus gains faith in himself and in the world. The existential therapist helps the neurotic to experience these forms of transcendence.

Faith is endangered by those experiences which threaten existence. The existential therapist must make the patient face the inevitability of such insecurity. Man feels shaken in his faith when he contemplates the arbitrariness of life. With the loss of faith in God goes the loss of faith in a universal order which makes everything in the world, including the individual person's life, illness, and death, part of an acceptable plan.

As poor substitute for religious faith, man constructs a shaky faith in a superstitious framework, often leading to obsessional actions which he uses as an insurance against the inevitableness of his fate. The existential therapist must confront such a person with the need to accept the risks of life as uninsurable. The following is an example: A woman of forty-five had developed a phobia of coloured people. Her trouble dated back to the age of twelve when she imagined that she would have to die within a year. She conceived the idea that coloured people were in possession of a dark power over life and death, and she was terrified lest she offended this power. She could never be sure that a coloured person might take umbrage at any of her actions.

She received first treatment from a psychoanalyst who, following the libidinal Freudian theory, interpreted her fear of the dark colour as a guilt feeling in relation to her anal function, the darkness standing for the colour of her faeces. The existential therapist brought her face to face with the fundamental challenge that death and calamity cannot be avoided and that we have to bear these risks and have to forgo the idea of an insurance vested in any power.

Once the nature of the danger has been recognized, the person can hope to come to terms with it. The anxiety which is aroused by the facing of an inevitable and destructive fate and which brings about numerous neurotic symptoms may be greatly reduced through confrontation. Man is helped when facing fate and death by the experience of transcendence. The facing is itself a task which must be undertaken before such help can be expected.

When discussing Heidegger's phenomenology, his insistence that everybody has a duty to come to terms with the experience of death and nothingness was accepted. The existential therapist concurs with Heidegger's criticism of the attitude of the people who avoid the issue of their fate and 'acquiesed in the unuttered decree of the "they", [which] is indifferent tranquility as to the "fact" that one dies'.[5]

Far from being a faith-destroying experience, death can be faith-inspiring. It was felt to be thus by the woman who wrote to the doctor whose attendance to her dying friend she had witnessed:

> A spiritual experience can be so easily overshadowed by material things that I want to tell you at once how much you did for all of us who were devoted to Florence. It was as if you, Florence, the night nurse and I were conscious of something for which I have no words, and your life's work seemed to give the light for that knowledge. It was like a beacon lighting up a spiritual plane.

The following accounts of existential therapy illustrate further how people can benefit from being confronted with the inevitableness of their situation.

A woman of thirty-six had developed obsessional thoughts about her skin and was convinced that the pores on her face were too large and that her whole skin was getting wrinkled. She was asked by an existential therapist what large pores on her face and wrinkles meant to her. She answered: 'Getting old.' The therapist could thus face her with this problem.

A business man of sixty-six, who was on the point of retiring from a busy life, complained of very disturbed nights: he kept waking up feeling sad, tense, and restless. He could not understand these feelings and became more and more frightened of going to sleep. The explanation was found in several reveries: his father had become senile, and the patient was terrified of developing the same symptoms of advancing age. In a semi-hypnotic state he was given the chance of discussing his fears, found the strength to face them, and was able to sleep peacefully.

An LSD treatment frequently involves facing terrors of birth, nothingness, and death. A woman suffering from agarophobia felt, under the influence of this drug, that she was entering a tomb and later on that she was dying. She found the strength to face life – and death – and recovered.

Another woman, aged forty, had encountered the terror of death from her earliest years; her grandfather died when she was two and she then saw that her mother was very upset. When she was twelve years old, she witnessed her father's nearly fatal attack of coronary thrombosis.

At about the same time, she was told that her mother had nearly died during her own birth. During her first pregnancy she consulted a doctor on account of phlebitis and was informed that a blood clot might easily travel from her leg to her heart and kill her. This patient suffered from a frightening choking sensation for which she could not account. In several reveries, the therapist led her back to the various experiences of her past life which were related to choking and the significance of the symptom was discovered: it stood for dying. Her fear of death was frankly discussed, and she learned to live with this fear without escaping into neurotic symptoms.

Apart from having to face the inevitability of age and death, people have to face the inevitability of illnesses which do not yield to treatment or which take time to clear up. The following is an account of a depressive illness which had to be endured for several years:

> This illness is like an abyss into which I have been pushed by fate. I grope about in the darkness, I feel only rocks and there is no way back to life. I dig into my mind, looking for my guilt to explain my fate. I scream in terror, but there is no answer, only the despair of loneliness.

In the loneliness of her illness, this patient felt tempted to turn away from her fellow human beings, as she 'did not wish to see [her] own unhappiness reflected in their faces'; but because of the communication with her therapist she found the strength not to shut herself away in despair and to face her suffering.[6]

EVALUATION OF EXISTENTIAL PSYCHOTHERAPY

Did the depressed patient who had received existential treatment not make just a spontaneous recovery? What is the evidence of the efficacy of this therapy? What statistical results or follow-up studies are available to support the existentialist's claim that his approach makes any difference to the neurotic illness? Such questions may be expected from a critic who has been brought up in the scientific tradition of our age.

In his reply, the existentialist must take a stand upon his premise and must not let himself be drawn from the realm of ethics into the world of science. To the existentialist, neurosis is a moral phenomenon. A patient is understood in relation to his conscience, as potentially free.

To the scientific psychiatrist, neurosis is a scientific phenomenon, a disease process which follows a natural course. Any claim that a particular form of treatment can influence this course in any way favourably must be substantiated by statistical evidence.

An example of the scientific approach to the psychological treatment of neurosis is the paper by R. Giel, R. S. Knox, and G. M. Carstairs, entitled 'A Five-Year Follow-up of 100 Neurotic Out-patients'. These authors carried out an 'overall evaluation of change' in 100 cases of neurosis which had not received any psychotherapy, and found recovery or considerable improvement, leaving the patient only with 'minimal disturbance of adjustment', in 71 per cent of cases. They concluded that 'any new treatment for the neuroses must show better than 70% improvement before it can claim to represent a significant therapeutic advance'. Giel and his co-workers also stressed the need of investigating the rate of relapses.[7]

An existential assessment of psychotherapy does not employ statistics, as each patient is considered as an individual person. The aim of the treatment is not to correct social adjustment and a 'minimal disturbance of adjustment' would not be accepted as a criterion of a successful psychotherapy. As society often causes a person's inauthenticity, the existentialist expects such a patient to refuse to be 'adjusted'; but, on the other hand, he also expects him to face the legitimate claims of the community. Under no circumstances can the existentialist's treatment be of no significance, as it is based on his relationship with the patient who needs this communication for attaining the freedom of authenticity available to him and for his liberation of transcendence.

With regard to 'relapses', the existential therapist agrees with Karl Jaspers that 'there is no straight road leading to self-realization. . . The self is a living and infinite self and is never complete'.[8] The emphasis is not on the objective state of mind, but on the subjective experience. In spite of the regrettable negative element of suffering, a relapse can have its positive, experiential meaning. Time is not chronological, but lived time, and each moment has unique significance of which a person has to be aware and which may have to be faced. Therefore the scientist's critical questions are not relevant for the evaluation of the existential approach.

While the existential therapist is justified in refusing to submit to the critical examination of the scientist, he must be his own critic. Although he is entitled to uphold the certainty of his moral philosophy, he has to admit his personal fallibility; he may well be mistaken in the interpretations of his patients' experiences and in his assessment of their strength and motivation. As he interprets the patients' conscience, he needs special awareness of his own conscience and constant self-criticism.

Summary

Neurosis is a manifestation of the contemporary crisis of valuation, a universal, moral phenomenon. For its understanding, a moral philosophy must be found.

Traditional systems of ethics are inappropriate, as they are concerned only with the analysis of concepts, and not with the effects which the acceptance of these concepts has on their holder. The philosophies of existence provide the obvious choice because they have been formulated as the result of man's predicament, which they also reflect. As there are many and often contradictory existential interpretations, a choice must be made.

The accounts of Heidegger and Sartre of existence demand special attention since they have been applied to psychotherapy. Both these systems of thought must, however, be ruled out because of their ontological assumptions which contradict the idea of existential freedom. Frankl's logotherapy must be rejected on account of its inconsistencies. A personal existential ethic, incorporating important elements of the philosophies of Jaspers and Buber, offers the foundation for the understanding and treatment of sufferers from existential neurosis.

While the neurotic patient is helped by the deterministic scientific knowledge of 'organic' and genetic psychiatry, and by various psychological and sociological assessments, he is harmed by the unfounded claims of alleged scientific personality theories and by such deterministic presumptions as are expressed in the various forms of scientism, phenomenologism, and in secular humanism.

The exclusive reliance on rationalism, evident in these abuses of the application of the ratio, must be abandoned, and irrationalism must be granted a place so that man can gain faith in his own potentialities and can overcome his existential neurosis.

Postscript

A medically-orientated system of ethics opens up a new perspective in contemporary thought. It implies a criticism of many works of modern art, literature, and philosophy which give expression to man's revolt against the senselessness of his existence, but which also sabotage any chance of a successful revolution.

A recent review of contemporary literature by Ihab Hassan, entitled 'The Literature of Silence' illustrates the situation.[1] Art is said to 'contain an element of danger or even subversion'. According to Lawrence Durrell, it may even 'by its very nature' be an outrage. The writer of the article concludes that 'a particular genre of modern literature seems to vindicate Durrell's view; it constantly touches on the experience which awes him. That experience is one of metaphysical revolt: Ahab striking the sun if it insulted him, or Ivan Karamazov returning his life-ticket to God'.

The writer of the review agrees with this message but also with its anti-therapeutic effects when he says: 'It is metaphysical revolt and at the same time metaphysical surrender, which is the desire for nothingness: "the cry of the mind exhausted by its own rebellion", as Camus put it. In outrage, then, the very being of man is put on trial. What ensues is a dialectic of violence, demonic action and demonic reaction compressed into a terrible unity which becomes finally a naught.'

While one realizes that the authors of this type of literature have expressed their experience truly, and while their art should be criticized only from an artistic point of view, one must protest against their implied claim of an objective, true assessment of man. Hassan, in his review, recommends that the perplexity of modern man should be faced and he asks for 'radical solutions' which should not turn out to be 'radical dissolutions'.

A novelist and a critic of literature cannot be expected to find a remedy for the existential malaise. Psychiatrists, who have so far avoided the issue of modern man's predicament, must now face their professional duties in this field and not just join in the silence recommended by Ihab Hassan and by the protagonists of 'the literature of silence'.

References

Chapter 1

[1] Ryle, Anthony (1967). *Neurosis in the Ordinary Family.* London; Tavistock
[2] *Ibid.*, p. 128
[3] *Ibid.*, p. 101
[4] *Ibid.*, p. 88
[5] *Ibid.*, p. 136
[6] Ellis, Frank P. (1967). 'Psychoneuroses replace fevers and rheumatism.' *Med. News,* 3 November, p. 2
[7] Laurie, Peter (1967). *Drugs,* p. 15. Harmondsworth; Penguin
[8] Leading Article (1967). '. . . But in the U.S.A. they're taking it seriously.' *Med. News,* 3 November, p. 3
[9] 'Half adults are smoking.' *Med. News,* 23 June 1967, p. 9
[10] Leading Article (1964). 'Smoking and death.' *Br. med. J.* **1**, 193
[11] Report in *Medical News-Tribune* **2**, 20
[12] Sargant, W. (1967). 'More psychiatric patients in doctors' surgeries.' *G.P.* **4**, 1
[13] 'Non-barbiturates: addiction risks.' *Med. News,* 2 July 1965, p. 24
[14] Quoted in Laurie, Peter (1967). *Drugs,* p. 39, Harmondsworth; Penguin
[15] In a survey of neurotic illness, only those cases are usually included which fall into one of the recognized diagnostic categories. They amount to only a fraction of neurotically sick people, but even these figures are enormous. For instance, H. Gwynne Jones (1966) reported in *Progress in Mental Health* (Office of Health Economics) that 'looked at in terms of sickness absence alone, anxiety conditions, psychoneuroses and disorders of character, behaviour and intelligence are responsible for the loss of about 17 million working days in Britain each year'.

Chapter 2

[1] Ryle, Anthony (1967). *Neurosis in the Ordinary Family,* pp. 139–140, London; Tavistock

[2] Mowbray, R. M. and Timbury, G. C. (1966). 'Opinions on psychotherapy: an enquiry.' *Br. J. Psychiat.* **112,** 360

[3] *Ibid.,* p. 359

[4] *Ibid.,* p. 358

[5] Lewis, Sir Aubrey (1961). *Undergraduate Teaching of Psychiatry and Mental Health Promotion.* World Health Authority Technical Report Series, No. 208, quoted in Leading Article (1963). 'Undergraduate Teaching in Psychiatry.' *Br. med. J.* **2,** 576

[6] Lewis, Sir Aubrey (1963). 'Medicine and the affections of the mind.' *Br. med. J.* **2,** 1553

[7] *Ibid.*

[8] Nagel, Ernest (1967). 'The nature and aim of science.' In *Philosophy of Science Today,* p. 4, ed. by Sydney Morgenbesser, London; Basic Books

[9] *Ibid.,* p. 5

[10] *Ibid.,* p. 12

[11] *Ibid.,* p. 13

[12] Nagel, Ernest (1961). *The Structure of Science: Problems in the Logic of Scientific Explanation,* p. 77, London; Routledge and Kegan Paul

[13] Eysenck, H. J. (1957). 'Drugs and personality, I. Theory and methodology.' *J. ment. Sci.* **103,** 128

[14] Hebb, D. O. (1954). 'The Problem of Consciousness and Introspection.' In symposium edited by J. F. Delafresnaye, *Mechanisms of Nervous Integration and Conscious Experience,* p. 405, Springfield, Ill.; Thomas

[15] See for instance, Karon, B. P. and Saunders, D. R. (1958). 'Some implications of the Eysenck-Prell study "The inheritance of neuroticism": a critique.' *J. ment. Sci.* **104,** 350–358

[16] The inclusion of biological psychology within genetic psychiatry is illustrated in a paper by Kallman, F. J. (1958). 'The use of genetics in psychiatry.' *J. ment. Sci.* **104,** 542

[17] Fenichel, O. (1945). *The Psychoanalytical Theory of Neurosis,* p. 582, London; Routledge and Kegan Paul

[18] *Ibid.,* p. 576

[19] Allport, G. W. (1967). 'The open system in personality theory.' In *Current Perspectives in Social Psychology,* p. 150, 2nd ed. Edited by P. Hollander and R. G. Hunt. London; Oxford University Press

[20] *Ibid.,* pp. 145–149

[21] Cantril, H. (1967). 'The human design.' In *Current Perspectives in Social Psychiatry,* pp. 61–66, 2nd ed. Edited by P. Hollander and R. G. Hunt. London; Oxford University Press

[22] *Ibid.,* p. 61

[23] Nagel, Ernest (1961). *The Structure of Science,* pp. 479–480, London; Routledge and Kegan Paul

[24] Taylor, Charles (1964). *The Explanation of Behaviour,* pp. 90–91. London; Routledge and Kegan Paul

[25] *Ibid.,* pp. 150–152

[26] *Ibid.,* p. 168

[27] Scadding, J. G. (1967). 'Diagnosis: the clinician and the computer.' *Lancet* **2**, 877

[28] See above p. 3

[29] Cartwright, Dorwin (1967). 'Achieving change in people: some application of group dynamics theory.' In *Current Perspectives in Social Psychology,* p. 525, 2nd ed. Edited by P. Hollander and R. G. Hunt. London; Oxford University Press

[30] *Ibid.,* pp. 525–526

[31] Jones, Maxwell (1968). *Social Psychiatry in Practice, The Idea of the Therapeutic Community,* p. 101, Harmondsworth; Penguin

[32] *Ibid.,* p. 30

[33] *Ibid.*

[34] Rees, T. P. (1957). 'Back to moral treatment and community care.' *J. ment. Sci.* **103**, 306

[35] Nagel, Ernest (1961). *The Structure of Science,* p. 530, London; Routledge and Kegan Paul

[36] *Ibid.,* p. 527

[37] *Ibid.,* pp. 522–523

[38] Angel, R. W. (1956). 'The concept of psychic determinism.' *Am. J. Psychiat.* **111**, 408

[39] Dilthey, Wilhelm (1927). *Understanding of Other Persons and Their Expressions,* pp. 122–123, Translated by H. A. Hodges (1944). *Wilhelm Dilthey.* London; Kegan Paul

[40] Jaspers, Karl (1962). *General Psychotherapy,* pp. 302–303, Manchester; Manchester University Press

[41] Ellenberger, Henri F. (1958). 'A clinical introduction to psychiatric phenomenology and existential analysis.' In *Existence, A New Dimension in Psychiatry and Psychology,* p. 100, edited by Rollo May, Ernest Angel, and Henri F. Ellenberger. New York; Basic Books

[42] *Ibid.*

[43] *Ibid.,* p. 106–107

[44] *Ibid.,* p. 103

[45] For a detailed epistemological discussion of the nature of the psyche and of the implications for a science of the mind see Ledermann, E. K. (1970). *Philosophy and Medicine.* London; Tavistock Publications and Philadelphia, J. B. Lippincott Co.

Chapter 3

[1] Jung, C. G. (1945). *Modern Man in Search of a Soul,* p. 70, London; Routledge and Kegan Paul

[2] Frankl, Viktor E. (1961). 'Basic concepts of logotherapy.' *Confinia Psychiat.* **4**, 99

[3] Frankl, Viktor E. (1960). 'Beyond self-actualization and self-expression.' *J. Existential Psychiatry* **1**, 10
[4] McInnes, D. R. G. (1963). 'Present trends in psychiatric treatment.' *Br. med. J.* **2**, 306
[5] Mannheim, Karl (1945). *Diagnosis of Our Time: Wartime Essays of a Sociologist.* 3rd ed. London; Routledge and Kegan Paul
[6] *Ibid.*, p. 1
[7] Dubos, R. (1959). *Mirage of Health, Utopias, Progress and Biological Change,* p. 167. London; George Allen & Unwin
[8] *Ibid.*
[9] *Ibid.*, p. 168
[10] Mannheim, Karl (1945). *Diagnosis of Our Time: Wartime Essays of a Sociologist,* p. 25, 3rd ed. London; Routledge and Kegan Paul
[11] *Ibid.*
[12] Russell, Bertrand (1946). *History of Western Philosophy,* p. 807, London; George Allen & Unwin
[13] For a summary of the main moral theories see for instance Hill, T. E. (1950). *Contemporary Ethical Theories.* New York; Macmillan
[14] Hindson, M. T. (1953). 'Religious humanism.' *Plain View* **8**, 74
[15] *Ibid.*, p. 71
[16] Whyte, Lance L. (1947). 'Science and human understanding.' *Listener,* 17 July, p. 99
[17] Fromm, Erich. (1949). *Man for Himself. An Enquiry into the Psychology of Ethics,* pp. 158, 160, London; Routledge and Kegan Paul
[18] *Ibid.*, p. 191
[19] *Ibid.*, p. 181
[20] *Ibid.*, pp. 186–189
[21] *Ibid.*, pp. 218–224
[22] *Ibid.*, p. 225
[23] *Ibid.*, p. 160
[24] Austin, Jean (1968). 'Pleasure and happiness.' *Philosophy* **42**, 53
[25] Frankl, Viktor E. (1960). 'Existential analysis and logotherapy.' *Surgo,* Candlemas, p. 1
[26] Frankl, Viktor E. (1961). 'Basic concepts of logotherapy.' *Confinia Psychait.* **4**, 101
[27] *Ibid.*, pp. 102–103
[28] Frankl, Viktor E. (1954). 'The concept of man in psychotherapy.' *Proc. R. Soc. Med.* **47**, 976–977
[29] Frankl, Viktor E. (1960). 'Existential analysis and logotherapy.' *Surgo,* Candlemas, p. 6
[30] Frankl, Viktor E. (1960). 'Beyond self-actualization and self-expression.' *J. Existential Psychiatry* **1**, 11
[31] *Ibid.*, p. 13
[32] *Ibid.*, p. 17

[33] Frankl, Viktor E. (1956). *Theorie und Therapie der Neurosen Einführung in Logotherapie und Existenzanalyse,* p. 95–96, Wien–Innsbruck, Urban & Schwarzenberg
[34] Frankl, Viktor E. (1960). 'Paradoxical intention: a logotherapeutic technique.' *Am. J. Psychother.* **14**, 522
[35] Frankl, Viktor E. (1960). 'Beyond self-actualization and self-expression.' *J. Existential Psychiatry* **1**, 10
[36] Frankl, Viktor E. (1960). *Theorie und Therapie der Neurosen Einführung in Logotherapie und Existenzanalyse,* p. 126, Wien–Innsbruck, Urban & Schwarzenberg
[37] See for instance Frankl, Viktor E. (1960). 'Existential analysis and logotherapy.' *Surgo,* Candlemas, p. 4
[38] Frankl accepts existential analysis as a basis for his logotherapy.
[39] Frankl, Viktor E. (1960). 'Beyond self-actualization and self-expression.' *J. Existential Psychiatry* **1**, 13
[40] It is a powerful support for the personalistic ethical approach that psychologists have been unable to agree on a measurable, fixed self. See Wylie, Ruth C. (1961). *The Self Concept.* Lincoln; University of Nebraska Press
[41] Jaspers, Karl (1953). *The Origin and Goal of History,* p. 157, London; Routledge and Kegan Paul
[42] Jaspers, Karl (1963). *General Psychopathology,* p. 348, Manchester; Manchester University Press
[43] *Ibid.,* p. 353
[44] Foulquié, P. (1948). *Existentialism,* p. 49, London; Dennis Dobson Ltd.
[45] May, Rollo (1953). *Man's Search for Himself,* pp. 138, 139, London; George Allen & Unwin
[46] *Ibid.,* p. 139
[47] *Ibid.,* p. 140
[48] Bugental, J. F. T. (1965). *The Search for Authenticity: An Existential–Analytic Approach to Psychotherapy,* pp. 31–32, London; Holt, Rinehard and Winston Inc.
[49] *Ibid.,* pp. 41–42
[50] *Ibid.,* p. 60
[51] *Ibid.,* p. 61
[52] *Ibid.,* p. 277
[53] *Ibid.,* p. 281
[54] *Ibid.,* p. 275
[55] *Ibid.,* p. 323
[56] Jaspers, Karl (1949). *The Perennial Scope of Philosophy,* p. 65, New York; Philosophical Library
[57] *Ibid.,* p. 64
[58] *Ibid.,* p. 64–65
[59] *Ibid.,* p. 64
[60] Husserl, Edmund (1931). *Ideas: General Introduction to Pure Phenomenology,* p. 270, London; George Allen & Unwin

[61] *Ibid.*, pp. 246–247
[62] For an elucidation of the notion of Husserl's intentionality see, for instance, Mohanty, J. N. (1954). 'The "Object" in Husserl's phenomenology.' *Philosophy and Phenomenological Research* **14,** 343–353
[63] Husserl, Edmund (1931). *Ideas: General Introduction to Pure Phenomenology,* p. 240, London; George Allen & Unwin
[64] Merleau-Ponty, M. (1962). *Phenomenology of Perception,* p. xviii, London; Routledge and Kegan Paul
[65] Buber, Martin (1959). *I and Thou,* p. 30, 2nd ed. Edinburgh; T. T. Clark
[66] *Ibid.*, p. 34
[67] *Ibid.*, p. 28
[68] *Ibid.*, pp. 30–31
[69] *Ibid.*, p. 70
[70] *Ibid.*, p. 16
[71] Buber, Martin (1965). 'Elements of the interhuman.' In *The Knowledge of Man,* p. 79, edited by Maurice Friedman. London; George Allen & Unwin
[72] Foulquié, P. (1948). *Existentialism,* p. 56, London; Dennis Dobson
[73] *Ibid.*, p. 50
[74] Sartre, Jean-Paul (1959). *Nausea,* p. 163, New Directions Paperback; U.S.A.
[75] Sartre, Jean-Paul (1951). *Iron in the Soul,* p. 245, London; Hamish Hamilton
[76] Jaspers, Karl (1963). *General Psychopathology,* p. 345, Manchester; Manchester University Press
[77] Duncan-Jones, A. (1955). 'The notion of conscience.' *Philosophy* **30,**
[78] *Ibid.*, p. 134
[79] Schweitzer, Albert (1946). *Civilization and Ethics: The Philosophy of Civilization,* p. 252, 3rd ed. London; Adam & Charles Black
[80] Sartre, Jean-Paul (1948). *Existentialism and Humanity,* p. 52, London; Methuen & Co.
[81] *Ibid.*, p. 53
[82] Schweitzer, Albert (1946). *Civilization and Ethics: The Philosophy of Civilization,* p. 262, 3rd ed. London; Adam & Charles Black
[83] Buber, Martin (1965). 'Guilt and guilt feelings.' In *Knowledge of Man,* pp. 126–127, ed. by Maurice Friedman. London; George Allen & Unwin
[84] *Ibid.*

Chapter 4

[1] 'Hippocratic era ending says computer doctor.' *Intern. med. Tribune of Great Britain* **2,** 1

[2] The criticism is not directed against the use of the computer which co-ordinates relevant data obtained from the patient and elicited by the doctor, only against unwarranted reduction of the patient to these data.
[3] *Ibid.*, p. 12
[4] 'Computers should be used "For patient, not disease".' *Intern. med. Tribune of Great Britain*, **3**, 1
[5] Young, J. Z. (1964). *A Model of the Brain*, p. 6, Oxford; Clarendon Press
[6] *Ibid.*, p. 20
[7] *Ibid.*, p. 17
[8] Young, J. Z. (1966). *The Memory System of the Brain*, p. 19, London; Oxford University Press
[9] *Ibid.*, p. 24
[10] Young, J. Z. (1964). *A Model of the Brain*, p. 6, Oxford; Clarendon Press
[11] See for instance, Pucetti, R. (1967). 'On thinking machines and feeling machines.' *Br. J. Phil. Sci.* **18** (1); George, F. H. (1956). 'Discussion: thinking and machines.' *Philosophy* **32** (121); Ritchie, A. D. (1957). 'Discussion: could machines be made to think.' *Philosophy* **32**, (120); Clack, R. J. (1966). 'Can a machine be conscious?' *Br. J. Phil. Sci.* **17** (3)
[12] Gauld, Alan (1966). 'Could a machine perceive?' *Br. J. Phil. Sci.*, **17**, 51
[13] *Ibid.*, p. 55
[14] Platt, Lord (1967). 'Medical science: master or servant?' *Br. med. J.* **4**, 442
[15] Bridgman, P. W. (1959). *The Way Things Are*, p. 206, Cambridge, Mass.; Harvard University Press
[16] McLuhan, Marshall (1967). *Understanding Media, The Extension of Man*, p. 53, London; Sphere Books Limited
[17] *Ibid.*, p. 374
[18] *Ibid.*, p. 57
[19] Sargant, William (1969). 'The physiology of faith.' *Br. J. Psychiat.* **115**, 505–578
[20] *Ibid.*, p. 506
[21] Apart from the introduction of the critical (and the uncritical) mind in Sargant's account, any computer implies the admittance of a mind (or minds), as it has been designed, programmed, and is also maintained or repaired by mental efforts.
[22] *Ibid.*, p. 509
[23] Millar, W. Malcolm (1958). 'Hysteria: a re-valuation.' *J. ment. Sci.* **104**, 815, 816
[24] *Ibid.*, p. 818
[25] *Ibid.*, p. 819
[26] *Ibid.*, p. 820

27 Farber, Leslie H. (1966). *The Ways of the Will,* pp. 144–145, London; Constable
28 Sullivan, H. S. (1953). *The Interpersonal Theory of Psychiatry,* p. 37, New York; Norton
29 *Ibid.,* p. 133
30 See above, p. 16
31 Erikson, Erik H. (1965). 'Psychoanalysis and ongoing history: problems of identity, hatred and nonviolence.' *Am. J. Psychiat.* **122**, 246
32 The super-ego is not only concerned with the prohibition of sexual gratification, the authority of the parents and of the community; it is concerned with many aspects of life, with norms which have nothing to do with instincts.
33 Rogers, Carl R. (1961). *On Becoming a Person,* pp. 206–207, London; Constable
34 *Ibid.,* p. 215
35 *Ibid.,* p. 217
36 *Ibid.,* pp. 220–222
37 *Ibid.,* p. 224
38 Broad, C. D. (1944). 'Review of evolutionary ethics by Julian S. Huxley', *Mind* **53**, 366
39 Taylor, A. E. (1925). 'Philosophy.' In *Evolution in the Light of Modern Knowledge: A Collective Work,* pp. 434–435, London; Blackie
40 Darwin, Charles (1917). *The Origin of Species by Means of Natural Selection,* p. 402, London; John Murray
41 Darwin, Charles (1894). *The Descent of Man, and Selection in Relation to Sex,* p. 619, 2nd ed. London; John Murray
42 Freud, Sigmund (1950). *Totem and Taboo,* pp. 141–143, translated by J. Strachey. London; Routledge and Kegan Paul
43 Huxley, Julian S. (1961). 'The humanist frame.' In *The Humanist Frame,* p. 20, Ed. by Julian Huxley. London; George Allen & Unwin
44 *Ibid.,* p. 37
45 Waddington, C. H. (1961). 'The human animal.' In *The Humanist Frame,* p. 72, Ed. by Julian Huxley. London; George Allen & Unwin
46 *Ibid.,* p. 73
47 *Ibid.,* pp. 78–79
48 Teilhard de Chardin, Pierre (1959). *The Phenomenon of Man.* London; Collins
49 *Ibid.,* p. 291–292
50 Medawar, P. B. (1967). *The Art of the Soluble,* pp. 71–81, London; Methuen
51 Papanoutsos, E. P. (1959). 'Freedom and causality.' *Philosophy* **24** (130)
52 *Ibid.,* p. 194

53 Bultman, Rudolf (1955). 'The quest for meaning in history.' *Listener,* September 1955, p. 329
54 Walsh, W. H. (1958). *An Introduction to Philosophy of History,* pp. 20–21, London; Hutchinson University Library
55 *Ibid.,* p. 106
56 Jaspers, Karl (1953). *The Origin and Goal of History,* pp. 241–242, London; Routledge and Kegan Paul
57 Hegel, G. W. F. (1931). *The Phenomenology of Mind,* p. 41 (translator's Introduction), 2nd ed. London; George Allen & Unwin
58 *Ibid.,* p. 600
59 *Ibid.,* p. 27 (translator's Introduction)
60 *Ibid.,* pp. 27–28 (translator's Introduction)
61 *Ibid.,* p. 28 (translator's Introduction)
62 Popper, K. R. (1963). 'What is dialectic?' In *Conjectures and Refutations: The Growth of Scientific Knowledge,* pp. 326–327, London; Routledge and Kegan Paul
63 Sartre, Jean-Paul (1957). *Being and Nothingness: An Essay on Phenomenological Ontology,* p. 565, London; Methuen
64 *Ibid.*
65 *Ibid.,* pp. 66–67
66 Marcel, G. (1948). *The Philosophy of Existence,* p. 49, London; Harvill Press
67 Sartre, Jean-Paul (1957). *Being and Nothingness: An Essay on Pehnomenological Ontology,* pp. 271 and 375, London; Methuen
68 *Ibid.,* pp. 364 and 408
69 Sartre, Jean-Paul (1946). *In Camera,* p. 166, London; Hamish Hamilton
70 Laing, R. D. (1960). *The Divided Self: A Study of Sanity and Madness,* p. 49, London; Tavistock
71 Laing, R. D. and Cooper, D. G. (1964). *Reason and Violence: A Decade of Sartre's Philosophy, 1950–1960,* p. 46, London; Tavistock
72 *Ibid.,* p. 76
73 Laing, R. D. (1967). *The Politics of Experience and the Bird of Paradise,* p. 100, Harmondsworth; Penguin
74 Laing, R. D. and Cooper, D. G. (1964). *Reason and Violence: A Decade of Sartre's Philosophy, 1950–1960,* p. 119, London; Tavistock
75 *Ibid.,* pp. 119–120
76 Strasser, S. (1965). 'Phenomenologies and psychologies.' *Review of Existential Psychology and Psychiatry* **5,** 89
77 See above, p. 23
78 Strasser, S. (1965). 'Phenomenologies and psychologies.' *Review of Existential Psychology and Psychiatry* **5,** 89
79 Howard, D. (1966). 'Hallucination: a phenomenological analysis.' *Review of Existential Psychology and Psychiatry* **6,** 211–229

[80] *Ibid.*, p. 212. The true hallucination is said to be a spontaneous activity of the mind, not the result of an effort of will, whereas the pseudo-hallucination is traced to such an act.

[81] Laing, R. D. (1967). *The Politics of Experience and the Bird of Paradise*, p. 137, Harmondsworth; Penguin

[82] Husserl, E. 'Pariser Vortrage.' Quoted in Stephen Strasser (1965). 'Phenomenologies and psychologies.' *Review of Existential Psychology and Psychiatry* 5, 93

[83] See above, p. 39

[84] Roberts, D. E. (1959). *Existentialism and Religious Belief*, pp. 6–7, New York; Oxford University Press

[85] Buber, Martin (1914). 'With a monist.' In *Pointing the Way: Collected Essays of Martin Buber.* Ed. and Translated by Maurice S. Friedman, p. 27, New York and Evanston; Harper Torchbooks

[86] *Ibid.*

[87] Buber, Martin (1948). *Israel and the World*, p. 49, New York; Schocken Books

Chapter 6

[1] The community of the occupational therapy department and of the so-called community hospital, which was discussed as a form of social psychiatry in a previous chapter, can also serve the purpose of existential therapy. As the present discussion is concerned with the work of the existential therapist (who may of course co-operate with other members of a hospital) forms of treatment which involve other staff will not be discussed.

[2] Freud, Sigmund (1914). *On Dreams*, p. 30, London; William Heinemann

[3] *Ibid.*, p. 87

[4] See, for instance, Freud, Sigmund (1923). 'Remarks upon the theory and practice of dream interpretation.' In *Yearbook of Psycho-analysis, Volume I (1945)*, p. 21, London; Imago

[5] Adler, Gerhard (1948). *Studies in Analytical Psychology*, p. 35, London; Routledge and Kegan Paul

[6] *Ibid.*, p. 37

[7] *Ibid.*, 36

[8] The 'reverie' method is similar to L. R. Wolberg's dramatization treatment (described in his *Hypoanalysis* which was published in 1946 by William Heinemann, Medical Books), but it is much less restricted than Wolberg's technique, as his dramas are performed in a state of deep hypnosis which can be reached only by a minority of patients. The main difference, however, lies in the respective aims of the two therapies: Wolberg sets out to release repressed emotions, such as anger and aggression, the existential therapist wants to provide an opportunity of facing critical life situations and dealing with them in order to achieve more personal freedom.

[9] Berger, Milton Miles (1957). 'The use of films for mental hygiene.' *Intern. J. of Social Psychiatry* **3**, 110
[10] Cohen, M. M., Marinelle, M. J. and Back, N. (1967). 'Chromosomal damage in human leukocytes induced by lysergic acid diethylamide.' *Science* **155**, 1417–1419
[11] Hungerford, D. A., Taylor, K. M., Shagass, C., La Badie, G., Balaban, G. and Paton, G. (1968). 'Cytogenic effects of LSD25 therapy in man.' *J. Am. med. Ass.* **206**, 2287
[12] Eysenck, J. (1967). 'LSD: unsubstantiated claims not evidence.' *Med. News* (Book Reviews Supplement) 12 May 1967, p. 9 (Review of Masters, R. E. L. and Houston, J. (1967). *The Varieties of Psychedelic Experience.* London; Anthony Blond)
[13] Buber, Martin (1958). *I and Thou,* p. 70, 2nd ed. Edinburgh; T. & T. Clark
[14] *Ibid.,* p. 133
[15] *Ibid.*
[16] Senguin, C. A. (1962). 'Love and psychotherapy, the psychotherapeutic eros.' *Acta psychoth.* **10**, 187
[17] *Ibid.,* p. 189
[18] Buber, Martin (1965). *The Knowledge of Man.* Ed. by M. Friedman. London; George Allen & Unwin
[19] *Ibid.,* pp. 182–183
[20] *Ibid.,* pp. 178–179
[21] A patient who is judged as not having the strength of responding to the existential approach must be treated by non-existential therapy, for instance with drugs.

Chapter 7

[1] Fingarette, Herbert (1962). 'Real guilt and neurotic guilt.' *J. Existential Psychiatry* **3**, 146, 147
[2] Guntrip, H. (1961). *Personality Structure and Human Interaction: The Developing Synthesis of Psychodynamic Theory,* p. 407, London; Hogarth Press and Institute of Psycho-analysis
[3] Jaspers, Karl (1962). *General Psychopathology,* p. 303, Manchester; Manchester University Press
[4] *Ibid.,* p. 353. See above, p. 37
[5] *Ibid.,* p. 348
[6] *Ibid.,* p. 353
[7] Jaspers, Karl (1922). *Psychologie der Weltanschauunger,* pp. 240 *ff,* 2nd ed. Berlin; Julius Springer

Chapter 8

[1] See above, p. 40
[2] Fenichel, O. (1945). *The Psychoanalytic Theory of Neurosis,* p. 29, London; Routledge and Kegan Paul

[3] *Ibid.*, p. 30

[4] May, Rollo (1958). 'Contributions of existential psychotherapy.' In *Existence: A New Dimension in Psychiatry and Psychology,* p. 79, Edited by May, R., Angel, E. and Ellenberger, H. F. New York; Basic Books

[5] Heidegger, M. (1962). *Being and Time,* p. 298, London; SCM Press

[6] The facing of death and of dangers does not only form part of psychotherapy. Young healthy people can benefit from having to meet life-threatening experiences as the following account of an educational experiment demonstrates:

A group of adolescent boys, aged sixteen to twenty-one are first trained to be physically fit at the Outward Bound School in the high mountain wilderness of Colorado. Then each boy undergoes 'a solo survival trip during which the boy spends 48 hours alone in the wilderness. He carries with him a knife, a snare, a string and fishhook, salt, matches and nothing else. The other is a group experience. This involves climbing the top of a mountain, during the course of which all the skills of climbing, axemanship, rope-handling, and physical conditioning are put to the test. as is the co-operative, supportive emphasis between patrol members.' (Clifford, E. and Clifford, M. (1967). 'Self-concepts before and after survival training.' *Brit. J. clin. Psychol.* **6**, 241–242. Psychological tests, applied to the boys, demonstrated that this survival training resulted in an increase of 'feelings of self-worth and competence' (*ibid.*, p. 248).

[7] Giel, R., Knox, R. S. and Carstairs, G. M. (1964). 'A five-year follow-up of 100 neurotic out-patients.' *Brit. med. J.* **2**, 160–163

[8] Jaspers, Karl (1922). *Psychologie der Weltanschauungen,* pp. 240 and 413, 2nd ed. Berlin; Julius Springer

Postscript

[1] Hassan, Ihab (1967). 'The literature of silence.' *Encounter,* **28**, 72–82

Author Index

Subject Index